GASTRIC BYPASS COOKBOOK

Simple and Tasty Nutritious Recipes after Weight Loss Surgery

By

Hector Wiggins

Table of Contents

INTRODUCTION

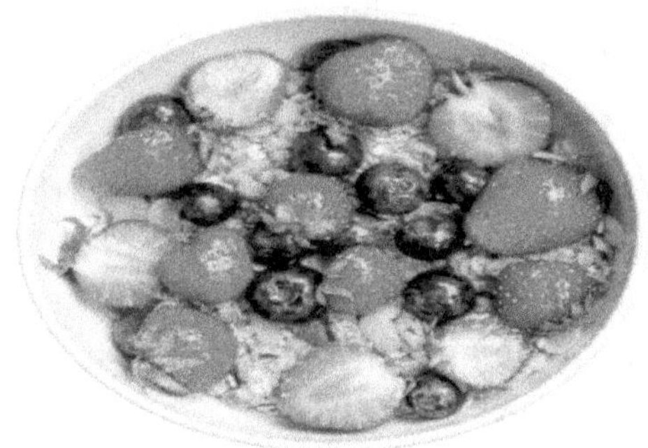

Welcome to the Gastric Bypass Diet's life-changing adventure. Regardless of whether you are contemplating gastric bypass surgery, are recuperating from the procedure, or have already had this transformative experience, this book serves as your all-inclusive resource for adopting a novel eating and lifestyle approach.

Many people make the very personal decision to have gastric bypass surgery in order to enhance their quality of life, mobility, and overall health. It stands for a dedication to assuming responsibility for one's health and wellbeing and starting along the road to long-term weight loss and management.

But the trip doesn't stop with the procedure. Actually, this is simply the start of a brand-new chapter in your life, one that calls for commitment, tenacity, and an openness to change. Adopting a specific diet designed to meet your body's particular post-surgery demands is essential to this journey.

The goal of the Gastric Bypass Diet is to fuel your body with the correct nutrients in the proper amounts to support recovery, encourage weight reduction, and prevent nutritional deficiencies. It is not simply about counting calories or limiting what you eat. It's about forming a better connection with food, becoming aware of your body, and learning to make thoughtful eating decisions.

We'll go deeply into the Gastric Bypass Diet's tenets in this book, arming you with the information, instruments, and resources you need to be successful on your path. Each chapter aims to provide you with the tools you need to take control of your health and adopt a wellness lifestyle, from comprehending the science underlying gastric bypass surgery to offering helpful advice on meal planning and preparation.

The basics of gastric bypass surgery will be discussed first, along with how it operates, who can benefit from it, and what to anticipate before, during, and after the operation.
It is essential to comprehend the reasoning behind gastric bypass surgery in order to make well-informed judgments regarding your health and to have reasonable expectations for the process that lies ahead.

We'll next get into the details of the Gastric Bypass Diet, dissecting its main elements and tenets. You'll discover the value of staying hydrated, eating a sufficient amount of protein, and getting the vitamins and minerals you need to maintain good health after surgery. We'll also go over typical problems and hazards that people on the Gastric Bypass Diet encounter, as well as solutions.

You'll discover lots of useful information in this book, such as meal planning, recipe ideas, advice on dining out, and strategies for handling social situations. We'll teach you how to prepare tasty, nutrient-dense meals that meet your nutritional requirements and help you achieve your weight reduction objectives, from filling breakfasts to satiating lunches and dinners.

The book's main message, nevertheless, may be one of empowerment. It's about giving you the tools you need to take charge of your health, make wise decisions, and live a lifestyle that puts vitality and wellbeing first. This book is here to help you every step of the way, regardless of where you are in your Gastric Bypass Diet journey or whether you're seeking for new inspiration and direction.

So let's go out on this road of change, resiliency, and revitalization together. The Gastric Bypass Diet is a compass that may lead you to a happier, healthier version of yourself.

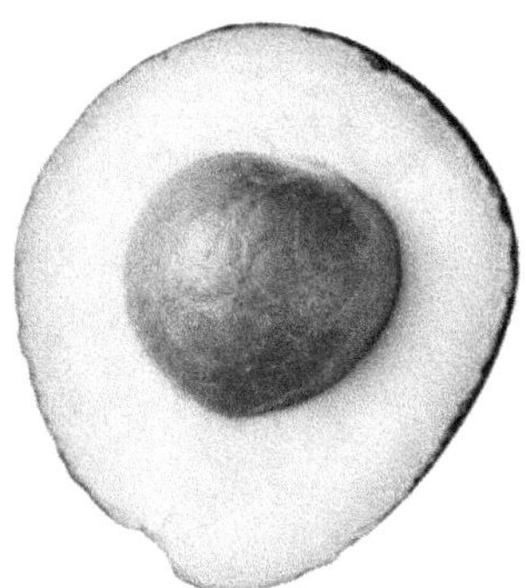

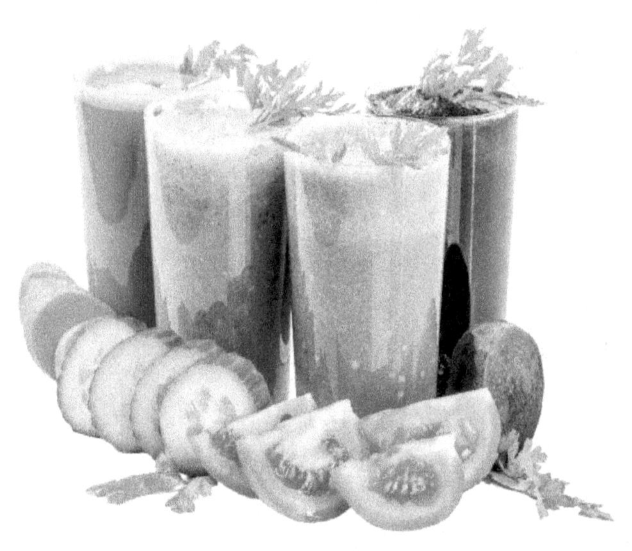

Understanding Gastric Bypass Surgery

The goal of gastric bypass surgery, commonly referred to as Roux-en-Y gastric bypass, is to assist people who are obese lose a considerable amount of weight in a way that will last. By changing the structure of the digestive tract, this revolutionary operation reduces food intake, decreases nutrient absorption, and modifies hunger and satiety signals. Those who are thinking about having gastric bypass surgery as a way to enhance their health and quality of life must comprehend the complexities of the procedure.

Anatomy of Gastric Bypass Surgery:
During gastric bypass surgery, the surgeon creates a small pouch at the top of the stomach, typically about the size of a walnut. This pouch serves as the new stomach, significantly reducing its capacity to hold food. The small intestine is then divided, and the lower portion is connected directly to the newly created stomach pouch, bypassing the rest of the stomach and the upper portion of the small intestine.

Mechanism of Action:
The primary mechanism of gastric bypass surgery involves restrictive and malabsorptive components. The smaller stomach pouch restricts the amount of food that can be consumed at one time, leading to feelings of fullness and satiety with smaller meals. Additionally, bypassing a portion of the small intestine reduces the absorption of calories and nutrients from food, further contributing to weight loss.

Benefits of Gastric Bypass Surgery:
Gastric bypass surgery offers numerous benefits beyond weight loss. Many individuals experience improvements in obesity-related health conditions such as type 2 diabetes, high blood pressure, sleep apnea, and joint pain. Additionally, the rapid initial weight loss following surgery can provide motivation and momentum for long-term lifestyle changes, including improved dietary habits and increased physical activity.

Considerations and Risks:
While gastric bypass surgery can be highly
effective, it is not without risks and considerations.
Potential risks and complications include infection,
bleeding, blood clots, gastrointestinal leakage, and
nutritional deficiencies. Additionally, the success of
gastric bypass surgery depends on a commitment to
lifelong dietary and lifestyle changes, including
regular exercise, mindful eating, and ongoing
medical monitoring.

Preparation and Recovery:
Prior to undergoing gastric bypass surgery,
individuals typically undergo a thorough evaluation,
including medical assessments, nutritional
counseling, and psychological evaluations.
Following surgery, patients will need to adhere to a
strict post-operative diet and gradually progress
from clear liquids to pureed foods and eventually
solid foods. Close follow-up with a
multidisciplinary healthcare team, including
surgeons, dietitians, and mental health
professionals, is essential for long-term success and
support.

A gastric bypass procedure can help obese people lose a large amount of weight in a sustained way, improve their general health, and live better. It is not, however, a one-size-fits-all remedy or a fast treatment. It is essential for anyone thinking about having gastric bypass surgery to comprehend the fundamentals, workings, advantages, and drawbacks of the procedure before starting on their path to better health and wellbeing. A better, happier future may be paved with gastric bypass surgery if the patient has the right information, preparation, and support.

Importance of Proper Nutrition Post-Surgery

Understanding the importance of proper nutrition post-surgery is paramount for individuals undergoing gastric bypass surgery in order to achieve long-term success and optimal health outcomes. After gastric bypass surgery, proper nutrition becomes more important than ever before. This is because the surgical alteration of the digestive system significantly impacts how the body absorbs and processes nutrients, making it essential to adopt a carefully planned and balanced diet to support healing, promote weight loss, and prevent nutritional deficiencies.

Enhanced Nutrient Absorption:
Gastric bypass surgery reduces the size of the stomach and bypasses a portion of the small intestine, leading to changes in the body's ability to absorb nutrients. With a smaller stomach pouch and altered intestinal anatomy, the capacity to absorb certain vitamins, minerals, and macronutrients may be compromised.

Therefore, consuming nutrient-dense foods and prioritizing high-quality sources of protein, vitamins, and minerals is crucial to ensure adequate nutrient absorption and prevent deficiencies.

Supporting Healing and Recovery:
Proper nutrition plays a pivotal role in supporting the body's healing and recovery process following gastric bypass surgery. Adequate intake of protein, vitamins, and minerals is essential for tissue repair, wound healing, and overall immune function. Protein, in particular, is crucial for muscle maintenance and repair, which is especially important during the initial stages of recovery when the body may be in a state of increased metabolic demand. By nourishing the body with nutrient-rich foods, individuals can promote optimal healing and minimize the risk of complications post-surgery.

Promoting Weight Loss and Maintenance:
One of the primary goals of gastric bypass surgery is to achieve significant and sustainable weight loss. Proper nutrition post-surgery is essential for supporting this goal by facilitating the body's ability

to burn fat, build lean muscle mass, and regulate metabolism. Consuming a balanced diet that emphasizes lean protein, whole grains, fruits, vegetables, and healthy fats can help individuals achieve and maintain a healthy weight over the long term. Additionally, adopting healthy eating habits and portion control strategies can prevent weight regain and promote lifelong success following surgery.

Preventing Nutritional Deficiencies:
Gastric bypass surgery can increase the risk of nutritional deficiencies due to reduced stomach capacity and altered nutrient absorption. Common deficiencies post-surgery may include vitamin B12, iron, calcium, vitamin D, and folate. These deficiencies can lead to a range of health complications, including anemia, osteoporosis, neurological disorders, and impaired immune function. Therefore, it is essential for individuals post-gastric bypass to work closely with healthcare professionals, including registered dietitians, to monitor nutrient status, identify deficiencies, and implement appropriate supplementation and dietary modifications as needed.

Improving Overall Health and Well-being:
Proper nutrition post-gastric bypass surgery is not just about preventing deficiencies or promoting weight loss—it's about optimizing overall health and well-being. A balanced diet rich in essential nutrients not only supports physical health but also contributes to mental and emotional wellness. Nourishing the body with wholesome foods can boost energy levels, enhance mood, improve cognitive function, and increase overall vitality. By prioritizing proper nutrition, individuals can maximize the benefits of gastric bypass surgery and enjoy a higher quality of life for years to come.

To sum up, the importance of proper nutrition post-gastric bypass surgery cannot be overstated. By nourishing the body with nutrient-rich foods, supporting healing and recovery, promoting weight loss and maintenance, preventing nutritional deficiencies, and improving overall health and well-being, individuals can optimize their outcomes and thrive following surgery. With the guidance of healthcare professionals and a commitment to lifelong dietary habits, individuals can embark on a

journey towards improved health, vitality, and
longevity.

How This Cookbook Can Help

This cookbook is a potent tool that uses the
transforming power of diet to assist and enhance
your gastric bypass journey. It is more than just a
compilation of recipes. Whether you're starting to
heal after surgery, dealing with dietary limitations,
or just looking for scrumptious and healthy meal
ideas, this cookbook is your all-in-one resource for
optimizing your gastric bypass experience.

Tailored to Your Needs:
One of the key ways this cookbook can help is by
providing recipes and meal plans specifically
tailored to the unique dietary needs of individuals
post-gastric bypass surgery. Each recipe has been
carefully crafted to align with the guidelines and
recommendations for gastric bypass patients,
ensuring that you're nourishing your body with the
nutrients it needs while supporting your weight loss
and health goals.

Variety and Flavor:

Gone are the days of bland and boring post-surgery meals. This cookbook is packed with a wide variety of flavorful and satisfying recipes that prove eating well after gastric bypass surgery can be both delicious and enjoyable. From hearty breakfasts to satisfying lunches and dinners, you'll find plenty of options to tantalize your taste buds and keep mealtime interesting.

Nutritional Balance:

Proper nutrition is paramount post-gastric bypass surgery, and this cookbook is dedicated to helping you achieve and maintain a balanced diet that supports optimal health and well-being. Each recipe is designed to provide essential nutrients, including protein, vitamins, and minerals, in appropriate portions to meet your dietary requirements and prevent nutritional deficiencies.

Practical Guidance:

In addition to mouthwatering recipes, this cookbook also offers practical guidance and tips to help you navigate the ins and outs of post-surgery eating. Whether you're learning how to portion control, meal prep like a pro, or make healthier choices when dining out, you'll find plenty of helpful advice to support your journey towards better health and wellness.

Empowerment and Inspiration:

Above all, this cookbook is about empowering you to take control of your health and embrace a lifestyle of wellness and vitality. By providing you with the tools, resources, and inspiration you need to succeed on your gastric bypass journey, this cookbook serves as a trusted companion and source of encouragement every step of the way.

Community and Support:
Finally, this cookbook is part of a larger community of individuals who are on a similar journey towards improved health and well-being. By sharing your experiences, tips, and recipes with others in the gastric bypass community, you can gain support, motivation, and inspiration to help you stay on track and achieve your goals.

CHAPTER ONE

The Basics of Gastric Bypass Friendly Cooking

Cooking after gastric bypass surgery requires a thoughtful approach to ensure that meals are both delicious and suitable for your dietary needs. The basics of gastric bypass friendly cooking encompass a range of strategies and techniques aimed at maximizing flavor, nutrition, and satisfaction while adhering to the guidelines and restrictions associated with post-surgery eating. Let's explore some essential principles and practices to help you navigate the world of gastric bypass friendly cooking with confidence.

1. **Emphasize Protein:**
Protein is essential for supporting healing, preserving lean muscle mass, and promoting satiety post-gastric bypass surgery. When cooking gastric bypass friendly meals, prioritize protein-rich

ingredients such as lean meats, poultry, fish, eggs, tofu, legumes, and low-fat dairy products.

Incorporating protein into each meal helps to ensure that you're meeting your daily protein requirements and staying satisfied between meals.

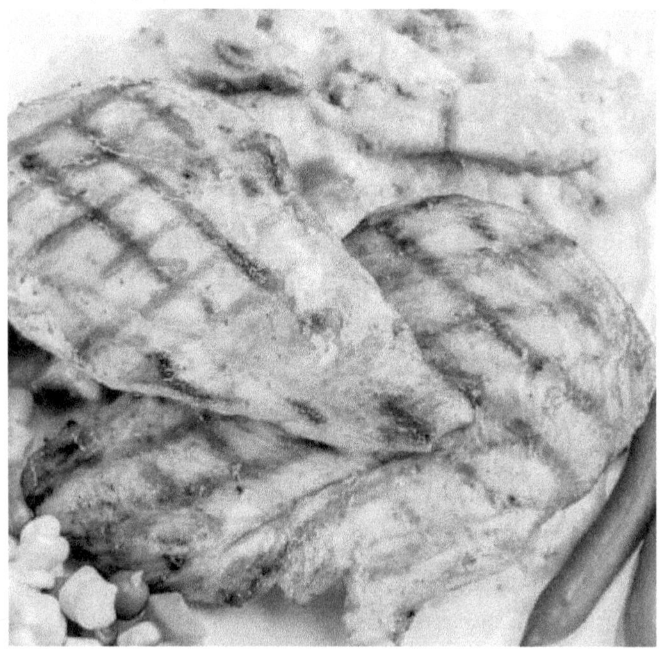

2. **Focus on Whole Foods:**

Whole foods are nutrient-dense and provide essential vitamins, minerals, and fiber to support overall health and well-being. When cooking after gastric bypass surgery, choose whole, minimally processed ingredients whenever possible. Load up on fruits, vegetables, whole grains, and legumes to add flavor, texture, and nutritional value to your meals. Experiment with a variety of colorful fruits and vegetables to create vibrant and satisfying dishes that nourish your body from the inside out.

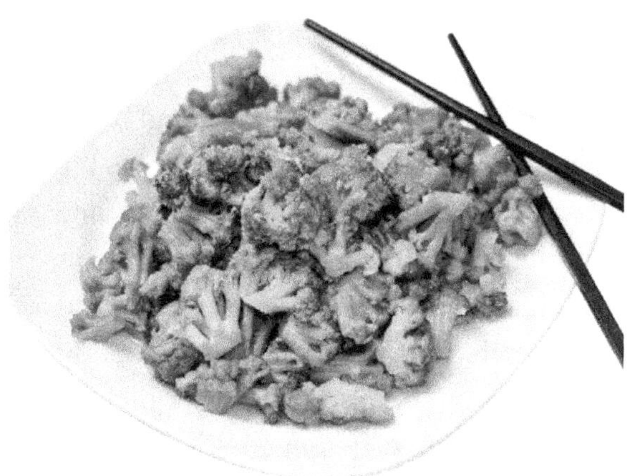

3. **Mindful Portion Control:**

Portion control is key to managing weight and preventing overeating post-gastric bypass surgery. When cooking gastric bypass friendly meals, pay attention to portion sizes and aim to create balanced and satisfying meals that provide the right amount of calories and nutrients for your needs. Use smaller plates, bowls, and utensils to help control portion sizes, and practice mindful eating by savoring each bite and listening to your body's hunger and fullness cues.

4. **Incorporate Healthy Fats:**

While it's important to limit added fats and oils post-gastric bypass surgery, incorporating healthy fats into your diet can provide flavor, satiety, and essential nutrients. Choose sources of healthy fats such as avocado, nuts, seeds, and olive oil to add richness and depth to your cooking without adding excessive calories or compromising your dietary goals. Experiment with different cooking methods, such as grilling, roasting, or steaming, to enhance flavor without relying on added fats.

5. Experiment with Flavorful Herbs and Spices:
Herbs and spices are powerful flavor enhancers that
can elevate the taste of gastric bypass friendly meals
without adding extra calories or sodium. Get
creative in the kitchen by experimenting with a
variety of herbs, spices, and seasonings to add
depth, complexity, and nuance to your dishes. From
aromatic herbs like basil, cilantro, and thyme to
bold spices like cumin, paprika, and turmeric, the
possibilities are endless when it comes to creating
delicious and satisfying meals that tantalize your
taste buds.

6. Prioritize Hydration:
Staying hydrated is essential for supporting
digestion, promoting healing, and preventing
dehydration post-gastric bypass surgery. When
cooking gastric bypass friendly meals, incorporate
hydrating ingredients such as broth-based soups,
fruits, vegetables, and herbal teas to help meet your
fluid needs throughout the day. Avoid sugary
beverages and excessive caffeine, which can

contribute to dehydration and undermine your
weight loss efforts.

These fundamentals of gastric bypass-friendly
cooking can help you prepare tasty, wholesome, and
filling meals that will help you achieve your
post-surgery wellness and health objectives. Your
body may be nourished and your path towards
better health and vitality fueled by a varied and
enjoyable diet that emphasizes whole foods, protein,
portion management, healthy fats, aromatic herbs
and spices, and plenty of water.

Guidelines for Cooking and Eating Post-Surgery Food

After undergoing gastric bypass surgery, it's crucial to adopt new cooking and eating habits that support your health, aid in recovery, and promote long-term success. These guidelines for cooking and eating post-surgery food serve as a roadmap to help you navigate the challenges and opportunities of your gastric bypass journey with confidence and ease.

1. **Start Slowly and Progress Gradually:**
In the immediate aftermath of gastric bypass surgery, your digestive system will need time to heal and adjust to its new anatomy. Begin with clear liquids and progress to full liquids, pureed foods, and eventually solid foods as directed by your healthcare provider. Take small, frequent meals and chew food thoroughly to aid in digestion and prevent discomfort.

2. Focus on Protein-Rich Foods:

Protein is essential for supporting healing, preserving muscle mass, and promoting satiety post-surgery. Incorporate protein-rich foods such as lean meats, poultry, fish, eggs, tofu, legumes, and low-fat dairy into your meals and snacks. Aim to include a source of protein with each meal to help meet your daily protein needs and support your weight loss goals.

3. Prioritize Nutrient-Dense Foods:

Option for nutrient-dense foods that provide essential vitamins, minerals, and fiber to support overall health and well-being. Load up on fruits, vegetables, whole grains, and legumes to add flavor, texture, and nutritional value to your meals. Choose whole, minimally processed foods whenever possible to maximize nutritional intake and promote optimal digestion.

4. Monitor Portion Sizes:

In order to regulate weight and avoid overindulging after surgery, portion control is essential. Observe serving sizes and pay attention to your body's signals of hunger and fullness. To assist reduce portion sizes, use smaller bowls, plates, and utensils. Steer clear of mindless nibbling or grazing in between meals. Prioritize quality above quantity in preparing meals that are delicious, well-balanced, and contain the appropriate number of calories and nutrients for your needs.

5. Stay Hydrated:

Staying hydrated is essential for supporting digestion, promoting healing, and preventing dehydration post-surgery. Drink plenty of fluids throughout the day, aiming for at least 64 ounces of water or other calorie-free beverages daily. Sip fluids slowly between meals to prevent overfilling your stomach and diluting digestive enzymes. Avoid sugary beverages and excessive caffeine, which can contribute to dehydration and undermine your weight loss efforts.

6. **Practice Mindful Eating:**
Choosing food carefully, enjoying every mouthful, and paying attention to your body's signals of hunger and fullness are all parts of mindful eating. Chew your meal well and slowly to help with digestion and avoid pain. To increase pleasure and happiness when eating, keep your attention off of electronic devices like laptops, cellphones, and televisions and concentrate instead on the sensory aspects of the meal.

7. **Supplement Wisely:**
Gastric bypass surgery can impact the body's ability to absorb certain nutrients, making supplementation essential for preventing deficiencies. Work closely with your healthcare provider to determine which supplements are right for you and to monitor your nutrient levels regularly. Common supplements post-surgery may include vitamin B12, iron, calcium, vitamin D, and multivitamins.

Essential Kitchen Tools and Equipment

Cooking and preparing meals after gastric bypass surgery require a thoughtful selection of kitchen tools and equipment to streamline the process, facilitate healthy cooking practices, and support your dietary needs. Whether you're blending smoothies, chopping vegetables, or portioning meals, having the right tools at your disposal can make all the difference in your post-surgery culinary journey. Let's explore the essential kitchen tools and equipment for gastric bypass patients:

1. Blender or Food Processor:
A high-quality blender or food processor is a must-have for gastric bypass patients, allowing you to easily puree foods, blend smoothies, and create nutritious soups and sauces. Option for a blender with variable speed settings and durable blades to ensure smooth and consistent results. A food

processor with different blade attachments can also be useful for chopping, slicing, and shredding vegetables and fruits.

2. **Immersion Blender:**

An immersion blender, also known as a hand blender, is a versatile tool that allows you to blend soups, sauces, and smoothies directly in the pot or container. Its compact size and easy-to-use design make it ideal for quick and convenient meal preparation, especially when working with small batch sizes or limited kitchen space.

3. **Food Scale:**

After gastric bypass surgery, precise portion control is crucial for controlling weight and avoiding overindulgence. By precisely measuring items using a digital food scale, you can be sure that you're following your nutritional rules and ingesting the appropriate portion sizes. For extra convenience, look for a scale that has an easy-to-read display and a tare feature.

4. Measuring Cups and Spoons:

Measuring cups and spoons are indispensable tools for portioning ingredients and following recipes accurately. Invest in a set of durable, easy-to-clean measuring cups and spoons in various sizes to

accommodate a range of portion sizes and cooking needs. Option for stainless steel or plastic measuring utensils with clear markings for easy reading.

5. **Small Cooking Pots and Pans:**

Small cooking pots and pans are ideal for preparing single-serving meals or portion-controlled dishes post-surgery. Choose nonstick or stainless steel pots and pans with lids for versatile cooking options and easy cleanup. Look for compact sizes that fit comfortably on your stovetop and are compatible with your cooking preferences and dietary requirements.

6. **Portion Control Plates and Bowls:**

Portion control plates and bowls are designed to help you visualize and maintain appropriate portion sizes while eating. These specialized plates and bowls typically feature portioned compartments or markings to guide serving sizes for proteins, grains, vegetables, and fruits. Using portion control plates and bowls can help you practice mindful eating and prevent overeating during meals.

7. Sharp Knives and Cutting Boards:

A set of sharp knives and cutting boards are essential tools for safely and efficiently preparing fruits, vegetables, meats, and other ingredients. Invest in high-quality chef's knives, paring knives, and serrated knives for versatile cutting, slicing, and chopping tasks. Choose cutting boards made of durable materials such as wood, bamboo, or plastic that are easy to clean and sanitize.

8. Meal Prep Containers:

You can batch cook and prepare meals for the week by portioning and storing dishes in advance with the help of meal prep containers. To store your meals fresh and safe, look for BPA-free, microwave-friendly containers with tight-fitting lids. To make the most of the space in your freezer or refrigerator, choose stackable containers.

Stock your kitchen with these necessary appliances and supplies to ensure a successful gastric bypass procedure. Having the correct tools at your disposal may help you negotiate the opportunities and challenges of cooking and food preparation after surgery with confidence, ease, and creativity—from making smoothies to portioning meals and engaging in mindful eating.

Tips for Meal Planning and Preparation

The following comprehensive tips will help you navigate meal planning and preparation after gastric bypass surgery: Meal planning and preparation is an essential part of post-gastric bypass surgery care, allowing you to nourish your body with nutritious, balanced meals while managing portion sizes and adhering to dietary guidelines. Careful planning and preparation can also reduce stress, speed up the cooking process, and support your long-term health and wellness goals.

1. **Consult with a Registered Dietitian:**
Speak with a qualified dietitian or nutritionist with experience in post-gastric bypass nutrition before starting your meal planning adventure. They may provide you individualized advice, methods for organizing meals, and suggestions based on your

own dietary requirements, tastes, and objectives for losing weight.

2. **Focus on Protein:**

Protein is a critical component of post-gastric bypass nutrition, supporting healing, preserving muscle mass, and promoting satiety. Plan meals and snacks that prioritize protein-rich foods such as lean meats, poultry, fish, eggs, tofu, legumes, and low-fat dairy products. Aim to include a source of protein with each meal to help meet your daily protein requirements and support your weight loss goals.

3. **Option for Nutrient-Dense Foods:**

Choose nutrient-dense meals that include necessary vitamins, minerals, and fiber to promote overall health and well-being. In order to enhance the taste, texture, and nutritional content of your meals, load up on fruits, vegetables, whole grains, and legumes. To guarantee a wide spectrum of nutrients and phytochemicals, include a selection of vibrant fruits and vegetables.

4. **Plan Balanced Meals:**

When meal planning, aim to create balanced meals that include a combination of protein, carbohydrates, and healthy fats. Use the plate method or the MyPlate guidelines as a template for portioning your meals, filling half your plate with fruits and vegetables, one-quarter with protein, and one-quarter with whole grains or starchy vegetables.

5. **Batch Cook and Freeze Meals:**

Batch cooking is a time-saving method that includes preparing big quantities of meals ahead of time and portioning them into individual servings for future consumption. Think about preparing grains, veggies, and protein sources in bulk so they can be quickly reheated and combined into well-balanced meals all week long. Purchase resealable bags or freezer-safe containers to preserve meals in the freezer for extended periods of time.

6. **Use Portion Control Tools:**

You may precisely measure and portion your meals to aid with weight reduction and prevent overeating by using portion control equipment like measuring cups, spoons, and portion control plates. With the

with the help of these tools, portion out the right amounts of grains, veggies, and protein. Then, engage in mindful eating by savoring each mouthful and paying attention to your body's signals of hunger and fullness.

7. **Experiment with Flavorful Herbs and Spices:** The key to enhancing the flavor and diversity of your food without consuming more fat, salt, or calories is to use herbs, spices, and seasonings. Try varying the herbs and spices you use to make your food taste better. This will help you make enticing meals that will make you want to eat after surgery.

8. **Plan for Snacks:** Include nutritious snacks in your meal planning to help you feel satiated between meals and reduce grazing or mindless munching. To supply you energy and stave off hunger throughout the day, choose nutrient-dense snacks like Greek yogurt,

cottage cheese, almonds, seeds, fresh fruit, and veggie sticks with hummus.

CHAPTER TWO

Breakfast Recipes

After undergoing gastric bypass surgery, it's essential to prioritize nutrient-dense meals that support healing, promote weight loss, and prevent nutritional deficiencies. Breakfast is no exception, serving as a vital opportunity to fuel your body and kickstart your day with nourishing options. These breakfast recipes are carefully crafted to meet the unique dietary needs and preferences of gastric bypass patients, providing balanced meals that are rich in protein, fiber, vitamins, and minerals while being gentle on the stomach.

1. **Protein-Packed Breakfast Bowl:**

This breakfast bowl is a satisfying and nutrient-rich option that combines cooked quinoa or brown rice with black beans, diced avocado, tomatoes, fresh cilantro, and a splash of lime juice. Quinoa or brown rice provides a hearty base rich in fiber and

complex carbohydrates, while black beans contribute plant-based protein and additional fiber. Avocado adds healthy fats and creamy texture, while tomatoes and cilantro provide freshness and flavor. This breakfast bowl is versatile and customizable, allowing you to adjust the ingredients to suit your taste preferences and dietary needs.

2. Veggie Egg Muffins:

Egg muffins are a convenient and portable breakfast option that can be prepared ahead of time and enjoyed throughout the week. These veggie egg muffins are made with a simple mixture of eggs, diced bell peppers, onions, mushrooms, and spinach, seasoned with salt and pepper. The eggs provide high-quality protein and essential nutrients, while the vegetables add fiber, vitamins, and minerals. These egg muffins are baked in a muffin tin until firm and golden, making them perfect for on-the-go mornings or quick and easy breakfasts at home.

3. **Overnight Oats with Nut Butter:**

Overnight oats are a no-fuss breakfast option that can be prepared the night before and enjoyed cold or heated up in the morning. This recipe combines rolled oats with unsweetened almond milk, nut butter, chia seeds, mashed banana, and optional toppings such as sliced bananas, berries, nuts, and seeds. Rolled oats are a good source of fiber and complex carbohydrates, while almond milk adds creaminess without excess calories. Nut butter provides healthy fats and protein, while chia seeds add omega-3 fatty acids and additional fiber. This breakfast is customizable and can be adapted to suit your taste preferences and dietary needs.

4. **Greek Yogurt Parfait:**

Greek yogurt parfaits are a delicious and satisfying breakfast option that can be assembled in minutes. This recipe layers plain Greek yogurt with granola, mixed berries, honey or maple syrup, and chopped nuts for added crunch and flavor. Greek yogurt is rich in protein and probiotics, which support digestive health and promote satiety. Granola adds crunch and texture, while mixed berries provide sweetness and a burst of antioxidants.

Honey or maple syrup can be drizzled on top for added sweetness, while chopped nuts add protein, healthy fats, and crunch. This breakfast parfait is customizable and can be tailored to suit your taste preferences and dietary needs.

5. **Protein Smoothie:**

Protein smoothies are a quick and convenient breakfast option that can be customized to suit your nutritional needs and taste preferences. This recipe combines unsweetened almond milk, frozen mixed berries, banana, protein powder, nut butter, and optional spinach or kale for added nutrients. Unsweetened almond milk provides a low-calorie base, while frozen berries and bananas add natural sweetness and fiber. Protein powder boosts the protein content of the smoothie, while nut butter adds healthy fats and creaminess. Optional spinach or kale can be added for additional vitamins,

minerals, and antioxidants. This smoothie is
blended until smooth and creamy, making it a
satisfying and nutrient-rich breakfast option.

These breakfast recipes are designed to provide
gastric bypass patients with delicious, satisfying,
and nutrient-rich options to start their day on the
right foot. By incorporating protein-rich ingredients,
whole grains, fruits, vegetables, and healthy fats,
these recipes support optimal health, satiety, and
energy levels post-surgery. Whether you prefer a
hearty breakfast bowl, protein-packed egg muffins,
creamy overnight oats, indulgent yogurt parfait, or
refreshing protein smoothie, there's something for
everyone to enjoy. Feel free to customize the
recipes according to your taste preferences and
dietary needs, and enjoy a satisfying and nourishing
breakfast that sets you up for success throughout the
day.

Protein-Packed Breakfast Bowl

Making protein-rich meals a priority after gastric bypass surgery is crucial for fostering healing, preserving muscle mass, and encouraging satiety. A tasty and nutrient-dense alternative, this protein-packed breakfast bowl mixes healthful ingredients to give you a boost of energy and vigor throughout the day.

Ingredients:
1/2 cup cooked quinoa or brown rice
1/4 cup black beans, drained and rinsed
1/4 cup diced avocado
1/4 cup diced tomatoes
1 tablespoon chopped fresh cilantro
1 tablespoon lime juice
Salt and pepper to taste

Optional toppings: sliced green onions, salsa, Greek yogurt.

Instructions:

Cook Quinoa or Brown Rice: Prepare 1/2 cup of cooked quinoa or brown rice according to package instructions. Both quinoa and brown rice are excellent sources of protein, fiber, and essential nutrients, providing a hearty and nutritious base for your breakfast bowl.

Prepare Black Beans: Rinse and drain 1/4 cup of black beans to remove excess sodium. Black beans are a rich source of plant-based protein and fiber, which helps to promote feelings of fullness and satisfaction.

Dice Avocado and Tomatoes: Cube 1/4 cup of ripe avocado and 1/4 cup of fresh tomatoes into small pieces. Avocado adds healthy fats and creamy texture, while tomatoes provide sweetness and acidity, enhancing the flavor profile of the breakfast bowl.

Chop Fresh Cilantro: Finely chop 1 tablespoon of fresh cilantro to add a burst of freshness and herbal flavor to the breakfast bowl. Cilantro not only adds vibrant color but also offers antioxidant properties and micronutrients.

Assemble Breakfast Bowl: In a bowl, layer the cooked quinoa or brown rice with the black beans, diced avocado, diced tomatoes, and chopped cilantro. Drizzle with 1 tablespoon of lime juice for a tangy kick, and season with salt and pepper to taste.

Add Optional Toppings: Add more creaminess and nutrition to your nutrition-Packed Breakfast Bowl by customizing it with optional toppings like salsa, chopped green onions, or a dollop of Greek yogurt.

Use your imagination and try out various flavor combinations to find what suits your palate.

Enjoy Your Nutrient-Dense Breakfast: Sit down, savor each bite, and enjoy your Protein-Packed Breakfast Bowl. This satisfying and flavorful meal provides a balance of protein, carbohydrates, healthy fats, vitamins, and minerals to fuel your body and mind for the day ahead.

Benefits of the Protein-Packed Breakfast Bowl:

High-Quality Protein: The combination of quinoa, black beans, and avocado provides a significant amount of protein to support muscle repair, satiety, and weight management.
Healthy Fats: Avocado contributes heart-healthy monounsaturated fats, while also providing essential vitamins and minerals such as potassium, vitamin E, and folate.

Complex Carbohydrates: Quinoa and brown rice offer complex carbohydrates, which are digested slowly to provide sustained energy and prevent blood sugar spikes.

Fiber and Nutrients: Black beans, tomatoes, and cilantro add fiber, vitamins, and minerals to the breakfast bowl, supporting digestion, immune function, and overall health.

Veggie Egg Muffins

For individuals who have undergone gastric bypass surgery, finding convenient and nutritious breakfast options is key to supporting their health and weight loss goals. Veggie Egg Muffins offer a delicious solution, packed with protein, fiber, and essential nutrients to fuel your morning without compromising on flavor or convenience.

Ingredients:
4 large eggs
1/4 cup diced bell peppers
1/4 cup diced onions
1/4 cup diced mushrooms
1/4 cup diced spinach
Salt and pepper to taste

Cooking spray or olive oil for greasing muffin tin.

Instructions:

Preheat Oven: Preheat your oven to 350°F (175°C) and lightly grease a muffin tin with cooking spray or olive oil to prevent sticking.

Prepare Vegetables: Dice the bell peppers, onions, mushrooms, and spinach into small pieces. These colorful vegetables add flavor, texture, and essential nutrients to the egg muffins.

Whisk Eggs: In a large mixing bowl, whisk together the eggs until well beaten. Season with salt and pepper to taste.

Combine Ingredients: Add the diced vegetables to the beaten eggs and stir until evenly distributed. The combination of colorful vegetables provides a variety of vitamins, minerals, and antioxidants to support overall health and wellness.

Fill Muffin Tin: Pour the egg and vegetable mixture evenly into the greased muffin tin, filling each cup about two-thirds full. Be sure not to overfill to prevent overflow during baking.

Bake: Bake the egg muffins for 20 to 25 minutes, or until they are set and have a gently golden top, by placing the muffin tray in the preheated oven. To test whether a muffin is done, stick a toothpick into the middle; when it comes out clean, the muffin is done.

Cool and Serve: Once baked, remove the egg muffins from the oven and allow them to cool in the muffin tin for a few minutes before transferring them to a wire rack to cool completely. Once cooled, the egg muffins can be stored in an airtight container in the refrigerator for up to one week.

Benefits of Veggie Egg Muffins:

Protein-Rich: Eggs are a complete source of protein, providing all nine essential amino acids necessary for muscle repair and growth. Each egg muffin is packed with protein to support satiety and muscle health post-gastric bypass surgery.

Nutrient-Dense: The addition of colorful vegetables such as bell peppers, onions, mushrooms, and spinach adds vitamins, minerals, and antioxidants to the egg muffins. These nutrients support immune function, digestion, and overall well-being.

Portion-Controlled: Veggie Egg Muffins are portion-controlled, making them an ideal breakfast option for individuals who are mindful of their food intake post-surgery. Each muffin provides a balanced combination of protein, vegetables, and healthy fats to keep you satisfied and energized throughout the morning.

Convenient and Portable: Egg muffins are easy to prepare ahead of time and can be stored in the refrigerator for quick and convenient breakfasts on busy mornings. They are portable and can be enjoyed at home or on the go, making them a versatile and practical choice for gastric bypass patients.

Overnight Oats with Nut Butter

Overnight oats with nut butter offer a convenient and delicious breakfast option packed with protein, fiber, and healthy fats to fuel your morning without causing discomfort or digestive issues.

Ingredients:
Half a cup of rolled oats
Half a cup of unsweetened almond milk, or your favorite milk substitute
One tablespoon of nut butter (almond or peanut butter, for example)

One spoonful of chia seeds
half a mashed banana
Sliced bananas, berries, almonds, seeds, honey, or
maple syrup are examples of optional toppings.

Instructions:

Combine Ingredients: In a mason jar or airtight
container, combine the rolled oats, unsweetened
almond milk, nut butter, chia seeds, and mashed
banana. The rolled oats provide complex

carbohydrates and fiber, while the nut butter adds
protein, healthy fats, and flavor. Chia seeds add
additional fiber and omega-3 fatty acids, promoting
satiety and digestive health.

Mix Well: Stir the ingredients until well combined,
ensuring that the nut butter is evenly distributed
throughout the mixture. You can adjust the
consistency by adding more or less almond milk
according to your preference.

Refrigerate Overnight: Cover the mason jar or
container and refrigerate the mixture overnight,

allowing the oats to absorb the liquid and soften. The overnight soaking process helps to break down the oats and chia seeds, creating a creamy and pudding-like texture that is easy to digest.

Add Toppings: In the morning, remove the jar from the refrigerator and stir the mixture to combine. You can add additional toppings such as sliced bananas, berries, nuts, seeds, honey, or maple syrup for extra flavor and nutrition. Get creative and experiment with different combinations to suit your taste preferences and dietary needs.

Enjoy Cold or Heated: Overnight oats can be enjoyed cold straight from the refrigerator or heated up in the microwave for a warm and comforting breakfast option. Simply transfer the oats to a bowl and microwave for 1-2 minutes, stirring halfway through, until warmed to your liking.

Benefits of Overnight Oats with Nut Butter:

Balanced Nutrition: Overnight oats with nut butter provide a balance of carbohydrates, protein, and healthy fats, making them a satisfying and nutritious breakfast option for gastric bypass patients. The combination of rolled oats, nut butter, and chia seeds offers a steady source of energy to fuel your morning activities.

Digestive Friendly: The overnight soaking process softens the oats and chia seeds, making them easier to digest and gentler on the stomach post-surgery. Nut butter adds creaminess and flavor without overwhelming the digestive system, while mashed banana contributes natural sweetness and additional fiber.

Customizable: Overnight oats are highly customizable, allowing you to tailor the ingredients and toppings to suit your taste preferences and dietary needs. Whether you prefer almond or peanut butter, sliced bananas or berries, nuts or seeds, the options are endless for creating delicious and nourishing combinations.

Convenient and Portable: Overnight oats can be prepared ahead of time and stored in the refrigerator, making them a convenient and portable breakfast option for busy mornings or on-the-go lifestyles. Simply grab the jar from the fridge and enjoy a nutritious breakfast wherever you are.

Greek Yogurt Parfait

Gastric bypass patients require nutrient-dense meals that provide essential vitamins, minerals, and protein while being gentle on the stomach and promoting satiety. A Greek yogurt parfait offers a delicious and versatile breakfast option that meets these criteria, combining creamy Greek yogurt with granola, mixed berries, and optional toppings for a flavorful and nourishing meal.

Ingredients:

1/2 cup plain Greek yogurt

1/4 cup granola (choose a low-sugar option)

1/4 cup mixed berries (such as strawberries, blueberries, raspberries)

1 tablespoon honey or maple syrup (optional)

1 tablespoon chopped nuts (such as almonds, walnuts).

Instructions:

Layer Greek Yogurt: Start by spooning 1/4 cup of plain Greek yogurt into the bottom of a glass or bowl. Greek yogurt is a rich source of protein and probiotics, which support digestive health and promote satiety post-surgery.

Add Granola: Sprinkle 2 tablespoons of granola over the Greek yogurt layer. Choose a low-sugar granola option to keep added sugars to a minimum. Granola adds crunch, texture, and complex carbohydrates for sustained energy throughout the morning.

Layer Mixed Berries: Add 1/4 cup of mixed berries on top of the granola layer. Berries are rich in antioxidants, vitamins, and fiber, which support immune function, digestion, and overall health. Feel free to use a variety of berries such as strawberries, blueberries, and raspberries for a colorful and flavorful parfait.

Drizzle with Honey or Maple Syrup (Optional): For added sweetness, drizzle 1 tablespoon of honey or maple syrup over the mixed berries layer. Opt for natural sweeteners in moderation to control added sugars and enhance the flavor of the parfait.

Top with Chopped Nuts: Finish the parfait by sprinkling 1 tablespoon of chopped nuts over the top. Nuts such as almonds, walnuts, or pecans add healthy fats, protein, and crunch to the parfait, providing satiety and satisfying texture.

Repeat Layers (Optional): If desired, repeat the layers of Greek yogurt, granola, mixed berries, honey or maple syrup, and chopped nuts to create a multi-layered parfait. This adds visual appeal and texture variation to the breakfast dish.

Serve and Enjoy: Serve the Greek yogurt parfait immediately and enjoy the creamy texture, vibrant flavors, and satisfying crunch of each layer. Feel free to customize the parfait with additional toppings such as shredded coconut, dried fruit, or a sprinkle of cinnamon to suit your taste preferences.

Benefits of Greek Yogurt Parfait:

High-Quality Protein: Greek yogurt is an excellent source of protein, containing more protein per serving than regular yogurt. Protein is essential for muscle repair, satiety, and weight management post-gastric bypass surgery.

Probiotics for Digestive Health: Greek yogurt contains probiotics, which are beneficial bacteria that support digestive health and gut function.

Probiotics help maintain a healthy balance of gut flora and may alleviate digestive issues common after surgery.

Antioxidant-Rich Berries: Mixed berries provide a variety of antioxidants, vitamins, and minerals that support immune function, reduce inflammation, and protect against oxidative stress. Berries are also low in calories and high in fiber, making them an ideal fruit choice for gastric bypass patients.

Customizable and Versatile: Greek yogurt parfaits are highly customizable, allowing you to tailor the ingredients and toppings to suit your taste preferences and dietary needs. Whether you prefer crunchy granola, sweet berries, or nutty toppings, the options are endless for creating delicious and nourishing parfaits.

After gastric bypass surgery, you may have a filling, nutrient-rich breakfast that promotes your overall health and well-being by including Greek yogurt parfaits in your routine. As you start your post-surgery journey, these parfaits with protein-rich Greek yogurt, antioxidant-rich berries, and customizable toppings are likely to become a beloved morning tradition.

CHAPTER THREE

Lunch and Dinner Recipes

It's crucial to eat meals that are not only tasty but also rich in nutrients after gastric bypass surgery in order to aid in recovery, encourage weight loss, and preserve general health. With a focus on catering to the specific dietary requirements and tastes of gastric bypass patients, these lunch and dinner dishes offer well-balanced meals that are high in protein, fiber, vitamins, and minerals, easy on the stomach, and certain to satisfy.

1. Grilled Chicken Salad:

Grilled chicken breast: Lean protein source that is easy to digest and high in protein.
Mixed greens: Low-calorie, high-fiber base packed with vitamins and minerals.
Cherry tomatoes: Provides a burst of flavor and antioxidants.

Cucumber slices: Adds crunch and hydration to the salad.
Balsamic vinaigrette dressing: Light and flavorful dressing option to enhance the salad without excess calories.

2. Baked Salmon with Roasted Vegetables:

Salmon filet: Rich in omega-3 fatty acids and protein, supports heart health and muscle repair.
Seasonal vegetables (such as bell peppers, zucchini, and carrots): Colorful assortment of

vegetables packed with vitamins, minerals, and fiber.

Olive oil, garlic, and herbs: Simple seasoning to enhance the flavor of the salmon and vegetables.

Lemon wedges: Adds brightness and acidity to the dish.

3. Turkey and Vegetable Stir-Fry:

Ground turkey or turkey breast strips: Lean protein source that is easy to digest and versatile for stir-frying.

Assorted vegetables (such as bell peppers, broccoli, and snap peas): Provides color, texture, and nutrients to the stir-fry.

Low-sodium soy sauce or tamari: Adds savory flavor without excess sodium.

Garlic and ginger: Aromatic spices that enhance the flavor of the stir-fry.

Brown rice or quinoa: Whole grain options that add fiber and complex carbohydrates to the meal.

4. Lentil Soup with Spinach:

Lentils: Plant-based protein source that is high in fiber and nutrients, supports digestion and satiety.

Fresh spinach: Adds vibrant color and nutrients to the soup.

Carrots, celery, and onions: Aromatic vegetables that provide flavor and texture to the soup base.

Low-sodium vegetable broth: Provides depth of flavor without excess sodium.

Garlic and herbs (such as thyme and rosemary): Seasonings to enhance the taste of the soup.

5. Grilled Vegetable and Quinoa Salad:

Assorted grilled vegetables (such as eggplant, zucchini, and bell peppers): Adds smoky flavor and nutrients to the salad.

Cooked quinoa: Protein-rich whole grain that adds texture and bulk to the salad.

Feta cheese or goat cheese: Creamy and tangy cheese options that complement the flavors of the grilled vegetables and quinoa.

Balsamic vinaigrette dressing: Light and tangy dressing option to tie the salad together.

Benefits of Lunch and Dinner Recipes for Gastric Bypass Patients:

High Protein Content: Each recipe incorporates lean protein sources such as chicken, salmon, turkey, and lentils to support muscle repair, satiety, and weight management.
Fiber-Rich Ingredients: Colorful vegetables, whole grains, and legumes provide fiber to support digestion, regulate blood sugar levels, and promote feelings of fullness and satisfaction.

Balanced Nutrition: These recipes offer a balance of macronutrients (protein, carbohydrates, and fats) as well as micronutrients (vitamins and minerals) to support overall health and well-being post-surgery.
Gentle on the Stomach: The recipes are designed to be easy to digest and gentle on the stomach, minimizing discomfort and digestive issues commonly experienced after gastric bypass surgery.
Variety and Flavor: Each recipe offers a variety of flavors, textures, and ingredients to keep meals interesting and satisfying, preventing boredom and promoting adherence to dietary guidelines.

After gastric bypass surgery, you may enjoy tasty and nourishing meals that support your health and weight reduction objectives by adding these lunch and dinner dishes to your meal planning repertoire. These recipes, which emphasize high-protein foods, high-fiber veggies, and balanced nutrition, are certain to become mainstays in your diet following surgery and provide you the confidence and fulfillment you need to go on your path to better health and wellbeing.

Grilled Chicken and Veggie Skewers

Grilled chicken and veggie skewers offer a flavorful and satisfying meal option that is well-suited for individuals who have undergone gastric bypass surgery. Packed with lean protein, fiber-rich vegetables, and vibrant flavors, these skewers are easy to digest, gentle on the stomach, and provide essential nutrients to support healing and weight management. Here's a comprehensive look at this delicious recipe:

Ingredients:

Boneless, skinless chicken breast or thigh meat, cut into cubes: Lean protein source that is easy to digest and rich in essential amino acids for muscle repair and growth.
Assorted vegetables (such as bell peppers, onions, zucchini, cherry tomatoes): Colorful array of vegetables packed with vitamins, minerals, and fiber to support overall health and digestion.
Olive oil: Heart-healthy fat that adds moisture and flavor to the chicken and vegetables.

Garlic, herbs, and spices (such as garlic powder, paprika, oregano): Seasonings to enhance the flavor of the skewers without excess sodium or calories.
Lemon wedges: Fresh citrus flavor to brighten up the dish and add a burst of acidity.

Instructions:

Prepare Chicken and Vegetables: Cut the chicken breast or thigh meat into uniform cubes and chop the assorted vegetables into bite-sized pieces. This ensures even cooking and allows the flavors to meld together on the skewers.

Marinate Chicken: In a mixing bowl, toss the chicken cubes with olive oil, minced garlic, and a sprinkle of your favorite herbs and spices. Allow the chicken to marinate for at least 30 minutes to infuse it with flavor and tenderness.

Assemble Skewers: Thread the marinated chicken cubes and chopped vegetables onto skewers in alternating layers, creating colorful and flavorful skewers. Leave a small space between each piece to ensure even cooking on the grill.

Grill Prep: To avoid sticking, preheat your grill to medium-high heat after giving it a quick cleaning and light oiling.

Grill Skewers: Place the assembled skewers on the preheated grill and cook for 8-10 minutes, turning occasionally, or until the chicken is cooked through and the vegetables are tender and slightly charred.

Serve: Once cooked, remove the skewers from the grill and transfer them to a serving platter. Squeeze fresh lemon juice over the skewers for a burst of citrus flavor and season with additional herbs and spices if desired.

Enjoy: Serve the grilled chicken and veggie skewers immediately, either as a standalone meal or paired with a side salad, whole grain, or low-carb option for a complete and satisfying meal.

Benefits of Grilled Chicken and Veggie Skewers for Gastric Bypass Patients:

High Protein Content: Chicken breast or thigh meat provides a lean source of protein that is essential for muscle repair, satiety, and weight management after gastric bypass surgery.

Nutrient-Dense Vegetables: Assorted vegetables add vitamins, minerals, and fiber to the skewers, supporting overall health, digestion, and immune function post-surgery.

Gentle on the Stomach: Grilling the chicken and vegetables ensures tender and easy-to-digest skewers that are gentle on the stomach and minimize discomfort after surgery.

Customizable and Versatile: The recipe is highly customizable, allowing you to use your favorite vegetables and seasonings to create personalized skewers that suit your taste preferences and dietary needs.

Convenient and Portable: Grilled chicken and veggie skewers are portable and convenient for outdoor grilling, picnics, or meal prep, making them an ideal option for busy individuals or on-the-go lifestyles.

Turkey and Avocado Lettuce Wraps

Turkey and avocado lettuce wraps offer a delicious
solution, providing lean protein, healthy fats, and a
variety of vitamins and minerals without excess
carbohydrates or calories. These wraps are light,
refreshing, and packed with essential nutrients,
making them an ideal choice for gastric bypass

patients looking for a satisfying and nourishing meal option.

Ingredients:

Lean ground turkey or sliced turkey breast: A lean source of protein that is easy to digest and supports muscle repair and growth post-surgery.
Ripe avocado: Provides heart-healthy monounsaturated fats, fiber, and essential vitamins and minerals such as potassium and vitamin E.
Lettuce leaves (such as butter lettuce or romaine): Serve as a low-calorie and low-carbohydrate alternative to traditional wraps, adding crispness and freshness to the dish.

Assorted vegetables (such as tomatoes, cucumbers, bell peppers): Add color, flavor, and texture to the wraps while providing essential nutrients and antioxidants.
Olive oil, lemon juice, and herbs (such as cilantro or parsley): Create a light and flavorful dressing to enhance the taste of the wraps without excess calories or sodium.

Instructions:

Prepare Turkey: Cook lean ground turkey in a skillet over medium heat until browned and cooked through. If using sliced turkey breast, simply slice it into thin strips for easy wrapping.

Mash Avocado: In a bowl, mash ripe avocado with a fork until smooth and creamy. Add a squeeze of lemon juice to prevent browning and enhance the flavor of the avocado.

Assemble Wraps: Lay out lettuce leaves on a clean work surface and spread a layer of mashed avocado onto each leaf. Top with cooked turkey, sliced vegetables, and a sprinkle of fresh herbs.

Fold and Roll: Carefully fold the sides of each lettuce leaf over the filling, then roll it up tightly to create a neat and compact wrap. Secure the wraps with toothpicks if needed to hold them together.

Serve: Arrange the turkey and avocado lettuce wraps on a platter and serve them immediately, either as a standalone meal or paired with a side

salad, soup, or low-carb option for added variety
and satisfaction.

**Benefits of Turkey and Avocado Lettuce Wraps
for Gastric Bypass Patients:**

High Protein Content: Turkey provides a lean
source of protein necessary for muscle repair,
satiety, and weight management post-surgery.

Cardiovascular Health: Avocado contributes
heart-healthy monounsaturated fats and a creamy
texture to the wraps, which also helps with nutrition
absorption and cardiovascular health.

Low in Carbohydrates: Lettuce leaves serve as a
low-calorie and low-carbohydrate alternative to
traditional wraps or bread, making them suitable for
individuals following a reduced-carbohydrate diet
post-surgery.

Rich in Nutrients: Assorted vegetables provide a
variety of vitamins, minerals, and antioxidants to

support overall health, digestion, and immune function.

Light and Refreshing: Turkey and avocado lettuce wraps are light on the stomach, easy to digest, and refreshing to eat, making them an ideal option for individuals who may experience digestive issues or discomfort after surgery.

By incorporating turkey and avocado lettuce wraps into your meal planning after gastric bypass surgery, you can enjoy a delicious, satisfying, and nutrient-rich meal option that supports your health and weight loss goals. With lean protein, healthy fats, and crisp vegetables, these wraps are sure to become a favorite addition to your post-surgery diet, helping you navigate your journey to improved health and well-being with ease and enjoyment.

Quinoa and Black Bean Salad

Quinoa and black bean salad is a flavorful and versatile dish that is well-suited for individuals who have undergone gastric bypass surgery. Packed with plant-based protein, fiber, and essential nutrients, this salad provides a wholesome and satisfying meal option that supports healing, promotes satiety, and aids in weight management. With its vibrant colors, diverse textures, and robust flavors, this salad is sure to become a staple in your post-surgery meal rotation.

Ingredients:

Quinoa: A complete protein source that is rich in fiber, vitamins, and minerals, supporting muscle repair and overall health post-surgery.

Black beans: High in protein and fiber, black beans provide sustained energy, promote digestive health, and contribute to feelings of fullness and satisfaction.

Assorted vegetables (such as bell peppers, cherry tomatoes, red onions, cucumbers): Add color, crunch, and essential nutrients to the salad, enhancing its flavor and nutritional profile.

Fresh herbs (such as cilantro or parsley): Provide aromatic flavor and freshness to the salad, elevating its taste and appeal.

Olive oil, lime juice, and spices (such as cumin, chili powder, garlic powder): Create a zesty and flavorful dressing that ties the salad together and enhances its taste without excess calories or sodium.

Instructions:

Cook Quinoa: Rinse quinoa under cold water to remove any bitterness, then cook it according to package instructions until tender and fluffy. Allow the cooked quinoa to cool to room temperature before assembling the salad.

Prepare Black Beans: If using canned black beans, drain and rinse them thoroughly under cold water to remove excess sodium. If using dried black beans, cook them until tender, then allow them to cool before adding to the salad.

Chop Vegetables: Dice assorted vegetables into bite-sized pieces and chop fresh herbs finely. This ensures even distribution of flavors and textures throughout the salad.

Assemble Salad: In a large mixing bowl, combine cooked quinoa, black beans, diced vegetables, and chopped herbs. Toss gently to mix everything together evenly.

Prepare Dressing: In a small bowl, whisk together olive oil, lime juice, and spices to create a tangy and flavorful dressing. Adjust the seasoning according to taste preferences.

Dress Salad: Drizzle the dressing over the quinoa and black bean mixture, tossing gently to coat everything in the dressing. Ensure that all ingredients are evenly coated for maximum flavor.

Chill and Serve: Cover the salad and refrigerate it for at least 30 minutes to allow the flavors to meld together and the salad to chill. Serve cold as a refreshing and nutritious meal option.

Benefits of Quinoa and Black Bean Salad for Gastric Bypass Patients:

High Protein Content: Quinoa and black beans are both excellent sources of plant-based protein, providing essential amino acids necessary for muscle repair, satiety, and weight management post-surgery.

Rich in Fiber: The combination of quinoa and black beans offers a significant amount of dietary fiber, which supports digestive health, regulates blood sugar levels, and promotes feelings of fullness and satisfaction.

Nutrient-Dense: Assorted vegetables and fresh herbs add vitamins, minerals, and antioxidants to the salad, supporting overall health, immune function, and well-being.

Low in Calories: Quinoa and black bean salad is naturally low in calories and carbohydrates, making it a suitable option for individuals following a reduced-calorie or low-carb diet post-surgery.

Versatile and Customizable: This salad is highly versatile and can be customized with your favorite vegetables, herbs, and spices to suit your taste preferences and dietary needs.

After gastric bypass surgery, including quinoa and black bean salad in your meal rotation allows you to relish a tasty, fulfilling, and nutritious meal that aids your health and weight management objectives. With its blend of plant-based protein, fiber-filled components, and lively tastes, this salad is bound to be a regular feature in your post-operative eating plan, facilitating your path to enhanced health and wellness with simplicity and pleasure.

Salmon with Roasted Vegetables

Salmon with roasted vegetables is a nutritious and delicious meal option that is well-suited for individuals who have undergone gastric bypass surgery. Packed with protein, healthy fats, vitamins, and minerals, this dish offers a balanced combination of nutrients to support healing, promote satiety, and aid in weight management. With its vibrant colors, rich flavors, and diverse textures, salmon with roasted vegetables is sure to satisfy your taste buds and nourish your body post-surgery.

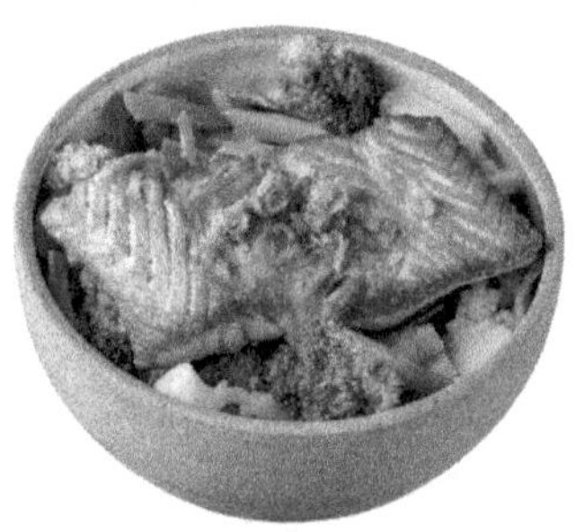

Ingredients:

Salmon filets: A rich source of omega-3 fatty acids and high-quality protein, salmon supports heart health, brain function, and muscle repair post-surgery.

Assorted vegetables (such as bell peppers, zucchini, carrots, and broccoli): Colorful and nutrient-dense vegetables provide vitamins, minerals, and fiber to support overall health and digestion.

Olive oil: Heart-healthy fat that adds moisture and flavor to the salmon and vegetables.

Garlic, herbs, and spices (such as thyme, rosemary, **garlic powder, paprika):** Seasonings to enhance the flavor of the dish without excess sodium or calories.

Lemon wedges: Fresh citrus flavor to brighten up the dish and add a burst of acidity.

Instructions:

Preheat Oven: Preheat your oven to 400°F (200°C) and line a baking sheet with parchment paper or aluminum foil for easy cleanup.

Prepare Salmon: Pat the salmon filets dry with paper towels and place them on the prepared baking sheet. Drizzle the salmon with olive oil and season with garlic, herbs, spices, salt, and pepper to taste.

Prepare Vegetables: Wash and chop assorted vegetables into bite-sized pieces. Arrange the vegetables around the salmon filets on the baking sheet, ensuring even spacing for even roasting.

Drizzle with Olive Oil: Drizzle the vegetables with olive oil and season with garlic, herbs, spices, salt, and pepper to taste. Toss the vegetables gently to coat them in the seasoning and olive oil.

Roast in Oven: Place the baking sheet in the preheated oven and roast the salmon and vegetables for 15-20 minutes, or until the salmon is cooked through and flakes easily with a fork, and the vegetables are tender and slightly caramelized.

Serve: Remove the salmon and roasted vegetables from the oven and transfer them to a serving platter. Squeeze fresh lemon juice over the salmon and vegetables for a burst of citrus flavor.

Enjoy: Serve the salmon with roasted vegetables immediately, either as a standalone meal or paired with a side salad, whole grain, or low-carb option for added variety and satisfaction.

Benefits of Salmon with Roasted Vegetables for Gastric Bypass Patients:

High Protein Content: Salmon is a rich source of high-quality protein, providing essential amino acids necessary for muscle repair, satiety, and weight management post-surgery.

Heart-Healthy Fats: Salmon is high in omega-3 fatty acids, which support heart health, reduce inflammation, and promote brain function and cognitive health.

Nutrient-Dense Vegetables: Assorted vegetables provide vitamins, minerals, and fiber to support overall health, digestion, and immune function post-surgery.

Low in Carbohydrates: Salmon with roasted vegetables is naturally low in carbohydrates, making it a suitable option for individuals following a reduced-carbohydrate or low-carb diet post-surgery.

Versatile and Customizable: This dish is highly versatile and can be customized with your favorite vegetables, herbs, and spices to suit your taste preferences and dietary needs.

Stir-Fried Tofu with Broccoli and Bell Peppers

Stir-fried tofu with broccoli and bell peppers is a satisfying and nutritious meal option that is perfectly suited for individuals who have undergone gastric bypass surgery. This dish is rich in plant-based protein, vitamins, and minerals, making it an excellent choice for supporting healing, promoting satiety, and aiding in weight management post-surgery. With its vibrant colors, savory flavors, and diverse textures, stir-fried tofu with broccoli and bell peppers is sure to delight your taste buds and nourish your body.

Ingredients:

Firm tofu: A versatile plant-based protein source that is low in calories and high in protein, essential for muscle repair and growth post-surgery.
Broccoli florets: Nutrient-dense cruciferous vegetable packed with vitamins, minerals, and fiber to support overall health and digestion.

Bell peppers (assorted colors): Colorful and flavorful addition that provides vitamins, antioxidants, and sweetness to the dish.

Garlic and ginger: Aromatic spices that enhance the flavor of the stir-fry without excess sodium or calories.

Low-sodium soy sauce or tamari: Adds savory umami flavor to the dish without excess sodium, perfect for seasoning tofu and vegetables.

Olive oil or sesame oil: Heart-healthy fat that adds richness and depth of flavor to the stir-fry.

Optional toppings: Sesame seeds, green onions, or cilantro for garnish and added texture.

Instructions:

Prepare Tofu: Drain the firm tofu and pat it dry with paper towels to remove excess moisture. Cut the tofu into bite-sized cubes or strips, ensuring uniform pieces for even cooking.

Stir-Fry Tofu: A tiny quantity of olive or sesame oil should be added to a big pan or wok that has been heated over medium-high heat. When the tofu cubes are golden brown and crispy on both sides, add them to the pan and cook for 5 to 7 minutes. After taking the tofu out of the skillet, set it aside.

Cook Vegetables: In the same skillet, add a little more oil if needed and add minced garlic and ginger. Stir-fry for 1-2 minutes until fragrant, then add broccoli florets and sliced bell peppers to the skillet. Cook the vegetables until they are tender-crisp, about 5-7 minutes, stirring frequently to prevent burning.

Combine Tofu and Vegetables: Once the vegetables are cooked to your liking, add the cooked tofu back to the skillet and toss everything together to combine. Cook for an additional 2-3 minutes to heat the tofu through and allow the flavors to meld together.

Season with Soy Sauce: Drizzle low-sodium soy sauce or tamari over the stir-fry, tossing to coat the tofu and vegetables evenly. Adjust the seasoning to taste, adding more soy sauce if desired for extra flavor.

Garnish and Serve: Transfer the stir-fried tofu with broccoli and bell peppers to a serving dish and garnish with optional toppings such as sesame seeds, sliced green onions, or chopped cilantro for added texture and freshness.

Enjoy: Serve the stir-fry immediately, either as a standalone meal or paired with a side of brown rice, quinoa, or cauliflower rice for a complete and satisfying dish.

Benefits of Stir-Fried Tofu with Broccoli and Bell Peppers for Gastric Bypass Patients:

Plant-Based Protein: Tofu is a rich source of plant-based protein, providing essential amino acids necessary for muscle repair, satiety, and weight management post-surgery.

Fiber-Rich Vegetables: Broccoli and bell peppers are both low-calorie, high-fiber vegetables that support digestive health, regulate blood sugar levels, and promote feelings of fullness and satisfaction.

Low in Calories: Stir-fried tofu with broccoli and bell peppers is naturally low in calories and carbohydrates, making it a suitable option for individuals following a reduced-calorie or low-carb diet post-surgery.

Heart-Healthy Fats: Olive oil or sesame oil adds heart-healthy monounsaturated fats to the dish, promoting cardiovascular health and aiding in nutrient absorption.

Customizable and Versatile: This dish is highly customizable and can be adapted to include your favorite vegetables, herbs, and spices to suit your taste preferences and dietary needs.

CHAPTER FOUR

Side Dishes and Snacks

Selecting the correct side dishes and snacks after gastric bypass surgery is crucial for sustaining optimal nutrition, encouraging healing, and assisting with weight reduction objectives. These foods should be tasty, high in nutrients, simple to digest, and provide a good mix of fiber, protein, vitamins, and minerals to keep you full and energetic all day. This is a thorough reference of snacks and side dishes designed specifically for those who have had gastric bypass surgery:

1. **Side Dishes:**

Steamed or Roasted Vegetables: Colorful vegetables such as broccoli, cauliflower, carrots, and Brussels sprouts are rich in vitamins, minerals, and fiber, making them ideal side dishes. Steam or roast them with a small amount of olive oil and seasonings for added flavor.

Mixed Greens Salad: A simple salad made with mixed greens, cherry tomatoes, cucumbers, and a light vinaigrette dressing is a refreshing and low-calorie side dish option. Add lean protein sources like grilled chicken, tofu, or hard-boiled eggs for extra satiety.

Quinoa or Brown Rice: Whole grains like quinoa or brown rice provide fiber and complex carbohydrates for sustained energy. Serve them as a side dish or base for protein-rich main courses such as grilled fish or tofu stir-fry.

Greek Yogurt with Fruit: Greek yogurt is high in protein and calcium, making it a satisfying side dish or snack option. Pair it with fresh berries, sliced bananas, or a drizzle of honey for added sweetness.

Cottage Cheese with Pineapple: Cottage cheese is rich in protein and low in carbohydrates, making it a filling and nutritious side dish or snack. Top it with pineapple chunks for a sweet and tangy flavor combination.

2. **Snacks:**

Hard-Boiled Eggs: Hard-boiled eggs are a convenient and portable snack option that is high in protein and low in calories. Enjoy them plain or seasoned with salt and pepper for added flavor.

String Cheese: String cheese is a convenient and portion-controlled snack option that is rich in protein and calcium. Pair it with whole grain crackers or fresh fruit for a balanced snack.

Nuts and Seeds: For long-lasting energy, a tiny handful of nuts and seeds, such as pumpkin seeds, walnuts, or almonds, offers good fats, protein, and fiber. Select unsalted kinds to reduce your consumption of sodium.

Vegetable Sticks with Hummus: Crunchy vegetable sticks like carrots, celery, and bell peppers paired with hummus make a satisfying and nutritious snack. Hummus provides protein and healthy fats while vegetables add vitamins, minerals, and fiber.

Protein Bars or Shakes: Protein bars or shakes are convenient options for on-the-go snacking, providing a quick and easy source of protein to keep you feeling full and satisfied between meals. Look for options with low sugar and high protein content.

Benefits of Side Dishes and Snacks for Gastric Bypass Patients:

Balanced Nutrition: Side dishes and snacks provide a balance of macronutrients (protein, carbohydrates, and fats) and micronutrients (vitamins and minerals) to support overall health and well-being post-surgery.

Sustained Energy: Nutrient-dense options like vegetables, whole grains, and protein-rich foods provide sustained energy throughout the day, preventing energy crashes and promoting stable blood sugar levels.

Portion Control: Pre-portioned snacks like hard-boiled eggs, string cheese, and single-serving yogurt cups help prevent overeating and support portion control, which is essential for weight management after gastric bypass surgery.

Convenience: Many side dishes and snacks are convenient and portable, making them easy to enjoy at home, work, or on-the-go, ensuring that you have access to nutritious options wherever you are.

Cauliflower Rice

Cauliflower rice has gained popularity as a low-carbohydrate alternative to traditional rice, making it an excellent choice for individuals who have undergone gastric bypass surgery. This versatile ingredient is not only easy to digest but also rich in essential nutrients, making it a valuable addition to the post-surgery diet. Whether used as a side dish, base for stir-fries, or as an ingredient in casseroles, cauliflower rice offers a satisfying and nutritious option for gastric bypass patients.

Nutritional Benefits:
Cauliflower rice is packed with nutrients while being low in calories and carbohydrates, making it an ideal choice for gastric bypass patients. Here are some key nutritional benefits:

Low in Calories and Carbohydrates: Cauliflower rice is significantly lower in calories and carbohydrates compared to traditional rice, making it suitable for individuals following a reduced-calorie or low-carb diet post-surgery.

High in Fiber: Despite being low in calories and carbs, cauliflower rice is rich in dietary fiber, which supports digestive health, regulates blood sugar levels, and promotes feelings of fullness and satisfaction.

Rich in Vitamins and Minerals: Cauliflower is a good source of vitamins C, K, and B vitamins, as well as minerals such as potassium and manganese, which are essential for overall health and well-being.

Antioxidant Properties: Cauliflower contains antioxidants such as beta-carotene, quercetin, and kaempferol, which help protect cells from damage caused by free radicals and oxidative stress.

Preparation Methods:
Cauliflower rice can be prepared in several ways, depending on personal preference and culinary needs. Here are some common methods:

Food Processor: Trim the cauliflower florets and pulse them in a food processor until they resemble rice grains. This method produces fine cauliflower rice that cooks quickly and evenly.

Box Grater: Use a box grater to grate the cauliflower florets into small rice-like pieces. This method results in slightly larger cauliflower rice grains, which may have a more rustic texture.

Frozen Cauliflower: Alternatively, you can purchase pre-riced cauliflower from the grocery store's frozen section, saving time and effort in the kitchen. Simply thaw the frozen cauliflower and use it as desired in recipes.

Usage Ideas:
Cauliflower rice can be used in a variety of dishes, offering a lighter and healthier alternative to traditional rice. Here are some creative ways to incorporate cauliflower rice into your post-surgery diet:

Stir-Fries: Use cauliflower rice as a base for stir-fries with lean protein sources such as chicken, tofu, or shrimp, along with colorful vegetables and savory sauces.

Grain-Free Pilafs: Create grain-free pilafs by sautéing cauliflower rice with aromatics like onions, garlic, and spices, then mixing in nuts, dried fruits, and herbs for added flavor and texture.

Casserole Fillings: Substitute cauliflower rice for traditional rice or pasta in casseroles, such as stuffed peppers, cabbage rolls, or baked dishes, for a lighter and lower-carb option.

Low-Carb Sushi Rolls: Roll up cauliflower rice with fresh vegetables, avocado, and protein sources like cooked fish or tofu to create homemade sushi rolls that are low in carbs and high in nutrients.

Stuffed Vegetables: Use cauliflower rice as a filling for stuffed vegetables such as bell peppers, zucchini, or mushrooms, mixing it with protein, cheese, and herbs for a satisfying and flavorful meal.

Cauliflower rice is a versatile and nutritious option for gastric bypass patients, offering a low-calorie, low-carb alternative to traditional rice that is rich in fiber, vitamins, and minerals. Whether used as a side dish, base for stir-fries, or ingredient in casseroles, cauliflower rice provides a satisfying and nourishing option that supports healing, promotes satiety, and aids in weight management post-surgery. With its versatility and nutritional benefits, cauliflower rice is sure to become a staple in your post-surgery diet, helping you enjoy delicious and satisfying meals while staying on track with your dietary goals.

Roasted Sweet Potato Wedges

Roasted sweet potato wedges are a delicious and nutrient-rich side dish that is well-suited for individuals who have undergone gastric bypass surgery. Packed with vitamins, minerals, and fiber, sweet potatoes offer a range of health benefits while providing a satisfying and flavorful addition to any meal. Whether enjoyed as a side dish, snack, or ingredient in salads or bowls, roasted sweet potato wedges are a versatile and nourishing option for gastric bypass patients.

Nutritional Benefits:
Sweet potatoes are a nutrient-dense root vegetable that offers several health benefits, especially for individuals following a gastric bypass surgery. Here are some key nutritional benefits:

Rich in Vitamins and Minerals: Sweet potatoes are high in vitamin A, vitamin C, manganese, and potassium, which support immune function, vision health, and electrolyte balance post-surgery.

High in Fiber: Sweet potatoes are a good source of dietary fiber, which promotes digestive health, regulates blood sugar levels, and helps prevent constipation—a common issue after gastric bypass surgery.

Low Glycemic Index: Despite their natural sweetness, sweet potatoes have a low glycemic index, meaning they cause a gradual rise in blood sugar levels, making them suitable for individuals managing diabetes or insulin resistance post-surgery.

Antioxidant Properties: Sweet potatoes contain antioxidants such as beta-carotene, which help protect cells from damage caused by free radicals and oxidative stress, supporting overall health and well-being.

Preparation Method:
Roasting sweet potato wedges is a simple and straightforward process that enhances their natural sweetness and creates a crispy exterior. Here's how to prepare roasted sweet potato wedges:

Preheat the oven to 425°F (220°C). Line a baking pan with parchment paper or aluminum foil for easier cleaning.

Prepare Sweet Potatoes: To get rid of any dirt or debris, give the sweet potatoes a thorough wash and scrub under cold water. Using a fresh kitchen towel, pat them dry.

Cut into Wedges: Using a sharp knife, carefully cut the sweet potatoes into wedges or fries of uniform size. Aim for wedges that are approximately 1/2 to 3/4 inch thick for even cooking.

Season with Spices: In a large mixing bowl, toss the sweet potato wedges with a small amount of olive oil or avocado oil until they are lightly coated. Season with your choice of spices, such as smoked paprika, garlic powder, cumin, or cinnamon, along with salt and pepper to taste.

Arrange on Baking Sheet: Arrange the seasoned sweet potato wedges in a single layer on the prepared baking sheet, ensuring that they are not crowded to allow for even browning.

Roast in Oven: After preheating the oven, place the baking sheet inside and roast the sweet potato wedges for 20 to 25 minutes, turning them halfway through, until the outsides are crispy and golden brown and the insides are still soft.

Serve and Enjoy: Remove the roasted sweet potato wedges from the oven and transfer them to a serving platter. Serve them immediately as a side dish or snack, garnished with fresh herbs or a sprinkle of sea salt, if desired.

For those undergoing gastric bypass surgery, roasted sweet potato wedges are a tasty and healthy alternative that provide a good mix of fiber, vitamins, and minerals in a tasty and filling meal. Sweet potato wedges are a flexible and healthful addition to your post-surgery diet, whether they are eaten as a snack, side dish, or component in other recipes. Roasted sweet potato wedges will quickly become a popular mainstay in your meal rotation thanks to its natural sweetness, eye-catching color, and multitude of health advantages. They'll also help you stick to your diet plan while chowing down on clean, delectable foods.

Guacamole with Veggie Sticks

Guacamole with veggie sticks is a delicious and nutritious snack option that is well-suited for individuals who have undergone gastric bypass surgery. Rich in healthy fats, vitamins, minerals, and fiber, guacamole offers numerous health benefits while providing a satisfying and flavorful dip for crunchy vegetable sticks. Whether enjoyed as a midday snack, appetizer, or light meal, guacamole with veggie sticks is a convenient and portable option for gastric bypass patients looking for a nourishing and satisfying snack.

Nutritional Benefits:
Guacamole and vegetable sticks offer a range of nutritional benefits, making them an excellent choice for individuals following a gastric bypass surgery. Here are some key nutritional benefits:

Healthy Fats: Guacamole is made primarily from avocado, which is rich in heart-healthy monounsaturated fats, known to reduce inflammation, support cardiovascular health, and aid in nutrient absorption.

Vitamins and Minerals: Avocado is a good source of vitamins C, E, K, and B vitamins, as well as minerals such as potassium, magnesium, and folate, which support overall health, immune function, and energy metabolism.

Fiber: Both guacamole and vegetable sticks are rich in dietary fiber, which promotes digestive health, regulates blood sugar levels, and helps prevent constipation—a common issue after gastric bypass surgery.

Antioxidants: Avocado contains antioxidants such as lutein, zeaxanthin, and beta-carotene, which help protect cells from damage caused by free radicals and oxidative stress, supporting cellular health and longevity.

Preparation Method:
Making guacamole with veggie sticks is quick and easy, requiring minimal ingredients and preparation time. This is how to make this healthy snack:

Prepare Guacamole:
Peel and pit ripe avocados, then place the avocado flesh in a mixing bowl.

Mash the avocado with a fork until smooth or leave it slightly chunky, depending on your preference. Add finely diced red onion, minced garlic, chopped cilantro, lime juice, salt, and pepper to the mashed avocado, mixing everything together until well combined.

Prepare Vegetable Sticks:
Wash and cut an assortment of colorful vegetables into sticks or strips, such as carrots, celery, bell peppers, cucumbers, and jicama.
Arrange the vegetable sticks on a serving platter or plate, ready to be dipped into the guacamole.

Serve and Enjoy:
Transfer the guacamole to a serving bowl and place it in the center of the platter of vegetable sticks.
Garnish the guacamole with additional chopped cilantro or a sprinkle of paprika for extra flavor and visual appeal.
Serve the guacamole with veggie sticks immediately, allowing everyone to dip and enjoy this nutritious and flavorful snack.

Guacamole combined with vegetable sticks is a nutritious and tasty snack choice that provides gastric bypass patients with a balanced intake of fiber, vitamins, minerals, and good fats in an easy-to-eat format. Eaten as a light meal, snack, or afternoon pick-me-up, guacamole with vegetable sticks is a tasty and nourishing approach to sate your appetite and replenish your body with necessary nutrients. This snack will quickly become a staple in your post-surgery diet thanks to its creamy texture, zesty taste, and crunchy toppings. It will keep you on track with your wellness and health objectives while providing you with enticing and nutritional food options.

Hummus and Whole Grain Crackers

Hummus and whole grain crackers make for a nutritious and convenient snack option that is perfect for individuals who have undergone gastric bypass surgery. This snack combines the creamy texture and savory flavor of hummus with the crunch of whole grain crackers, providing a satisfying and satisfyingly balanced snack that is rich in protein, fiber, vitamins, and minerals. Whether enjoyed as a midday pick-me-up, afternoon snack, or light meal, hummus and whole grain crackers offer gastric bypass patients a tasty and nourishing option to support their health and wellness goals.

Nutritional Benefits:
Hummus and whole grain crackers offer a range of nutritional benefits, making them an excellent choice for individuals following a gastric bypass surgery. Here are some key nutritional benefits:

Protein-Rich: Hummus is made primarily from chickpeas (garbanzo beans), which are a good source of plant-based protein. Protein is essential for muscle repair, satiety, and overall health, especially after gastric bypass surgery.

Fiber: Both hummus and whole grain crackers are rich in dietary fiber, which promotes digestive health, regulates blood sugar levels, and helps prevent constipation—a common issue after gastric bypass surgery.

Healthy Fats: Hummus contains heart-healthy fats from olive oil and tahini (sesame seed paste), which support cardiovascular health, reduce inflammation, and aid in nutrient absorption.

Vitamins and Minerals: Hummus and whole grain crackers provide a variety of vitamins and minerals, including vitamin E, vitamin B6, folate, iron, and magnesium, which support overall health and well-being.

Preparation Method:

Assembling hummus and whole grain crackers is quick and easy, requiring minimal preparation time. Here's the method for making this nutritious treat:

Select Hummus: Choose your favorite flavor of hummus, such as classic, roasted red pepper, garlic, or spicy. Alternatively, you can make your own hummus at home using canned chickpeas, tahini, olive oil, garlic, lemon juice, and spices.

Choose Whole Grain Crackers: Select whole grain crackers that are high in fiber and low in added sugars and sodium. Look for options made with whole wheat, oats, quinoa, or seeds for added nutritional benefits.

Assemble Snack: Spread a generous amount of hummus onto each whole grain cracker using a knife or spoon. Arrange the hummus-coated crackers on a serving platter or plate, ready to be enjoyed.

Garnish (Optional): Garnish the hummus with a drizzle of olive oil, a sprinkle of paprika, chopped fresh herbs, or a few toasted pine nuts for added flavor and visual appeal.

Serve and Enjoy: Serve the hummus and whole grain crackers immediately, allowing everyone to enjoy this wholesome and satisfying snack. Pair it with a glass of water or herbal tea for added hydration and refreshment.

Cottage Cheese and Fruit Bowl

One tasty and healthy snack choice designed specifically for those who have had gastric bypass surgery is a bowl of fruit and cottage cheese. This snack offers a gratifying and well-balanced choice to maintain post-surgery nutritional demands by combining the creamy texture and high protein content of cottage cheese with the inherent sweetness and micronutrients of fresh fruit. For gastric bypass patients, the cottage cheese and fruit bowl is a tasty and nutritious option that will fulfill their cravings and feed their bodies, whether it is consumed as a midday snack, breakfast substitute, or dessert.

Nutritional Benefits:
The cottage cheese and fruit bowl offer a plethora of nutritional benefits, making it an ideal snack for gastric bypass patients:

High Protein Content: Cottage cheese is rich in protein, which is essential for muscle repair, satiety, and overall health post-surgery. Protein helps support muscle mass and aids in recovery, making it an important component of the post-gastric bypass diet.

Low in Carbohydrates: Fresh fruit provides natural sweetness and vitamins without the excessive carbohydrates found in processed snacks or sweets. This makes the cottage cheese and fruit bowl a suitable option for individuals following a reduced-carbohydrate or low-glycemic diet post-surgery.

Rich in Vitamins and Minerals: Fresh fruit is packed with vitamins, minerals, and antioxidants that support immune function, cell repair, and overall well-being. Common fruits such as berries, melons, and citrus fruits are particularly rich in vitamin C, which aids in wound healing and collagen production post-surgery.

Healthy Fats: Cottage cheese contains some healthy fats, providing essential fatty acids that support brain health, hormone production, and nutrient absorption. Pairing cottage cheese with fruits like avocado or nuts adds additional healthy fats for sustained energy and satiety.

Preparation Method:
Creating a cottage cheese and fruit bowl is simple and requires minimal preparation time. Here's how to assemble this nutritious and refreshing snack:

Choose Cottage Cheese: Select your preferred variety of cottage cheese, such as low-fat, full-fat, or lactose-free, depending on your dietary preferences and tolerances. Opt for cottage cheese with no added sugars or artificial ingredients for a healthier option.

Select Fresh Fruit: Choose a variety of fresh fruits to complement the cottage cheese. Popular options include berries (strawberries, blueberries, raspberries), melons (cantaloupe, honeydew), citrus fruits (orange segments), kiwi, pineapple, and banana. Select fruits that are ripe and in season for optimal flavor and nutrition.

Prepare Fruit: Wash, peel (if necessary), and chop the fresh fruit into bite-sized pieces. Arrange the fruit in a bowl or serving dish, either mixed together or grouped by type for visual appeal.

Add Cottage Cheese: Spoon a generous portion of cottage cheese over the fresh fruit in the bowl. Use enough cottage cheese to provide adequate protein and creaminess to the snack, but adjust the portion size based on your individual dietary needs and preferences.

Garnish (Optional): For added flavor and texture, garnish the cottage cheese and fruit bowl with toppings such as chopped nuts (almonds, walnuts), seeds (chia seeds, flaxseeds), granola, or a drizzle of honey or maple syrup. Be mindful of portion sizes and added sugars when choosing toppings.

Serve and Enjoy: Serve the cottage cheese and fruit bowl immediately, either as a standalone snack or paired with a slice of whole grain toast or crackers for added variety and satisfaction. Enjoy the creamy texture of the cottage cheese paired with the juicy sweetness of the fruit for a delightful and nourishing snack experience.

CHAPTER FIVE

Soups and Stews

After undergoing gastric bypass surgery, it's crucial to follow a specialized diet to aid in recovery and ensure long-term success. Soups and stews are excellent options during the initial stages of recovery, providing essential nutrients while being easy on the digestive system.

Benefits of Soups and Stews:

Easy to Digest: Soups and stews are often blended or cooked until ingredients are soft, making them gentle on the stomach and easy to digest, which is particularly important after gastric bypass surgery.

Hydration: Many soups and stews have high water content, helping to keep patients hydrated, which is essential for healing and overall health.

Nutrient-Rich: By incorporating a variety of vegetables, lean proteins, and healthy grains, soups and stews can provide essential nutrients needed for recovery, such as protein, vitamins, and minerals.

Portion Control: After gastric bypass surgery, portion control is essential. Soups and stews allow for easy portion control, helping patients avoid overeating while still feeling satisfied.

Recommended Soups and Stews:

Chicken and Vegetable Soup: A classic option packed with protein from chicken and an array of nutrients from vegetables like carrots, celery, and spinach. This comforting dish is easy to digest and can be made in large batches for convenience.

Lentil Stew: Lentils are rich in protein and fiber, making them an excellent choice for post-surgery recovery. Combine with carrots, onions, and tomatoes for a hearty and nutritious stew.

Butternut Squash Soup: Creamy butternut squash soup is both soothing and nutritious. It's loaded with vitamins A and C, as well as fiber, making it a satisfying option for patients recovering from gastric bypass surgery.

Turkey Chili: Lean ground turkey combined with beans and spices creates a flavorful and protein-packed chili. It's a great option for those craving something with a bit of heat while still adhering to the post-surgery diet guidelines.

Vegetable Broth: For patients in the early stages of recovery, a simple vegetable broth can provide hydration and essential nutrients without overwhelming the digestive system. It's also versatile, allowing for customization with herbs and spices.

Chicken and Vegetable Soup

Chicken and Vegetable Soup tailored for individuals who have undergone gastric bypass surgery needs to be nutrient-dense, low in fat, and easy to digest. Here's a detailed recipe:

Ingredients:
2 cups of low-sodium chicken broth
1 cup of cooked, shredded chicken breast (skinless)
1 cup of mixed vegetables (such as carrots, celery, zucchini, and spinach), chopped finely
1/2 cup of finely diced onion
2 cloves of garlic, minced
1 teaspoon of olive oil
Salt and pepper to taste
Optional: herbs like thyme or parsley for flavor.

Instructions:
Warm up the olive oil in a big saucepan over medium heat. Add minced garlic and diced onion. Sauté until onions are translucent.
Add mixed vegetables to the pot and cook for a few minutes until they start to soften.

Pour in the low-sodium chicken broth and bring to a gentle boil.
Once the broth is boiling, reduce the heat to low and add the shredded chicken breast.
Simmer the soup for about 10-15 minutes, allowing the flavors to meld together.
Season with salt, pepper, and any additional herbs you prefer.
If needed, taste the soup and adjust the seasoning.
Serve the soup hot and enjoy!

This soup is packed with protein from the chicken breast and nutrients from the mixed vegetables. It's low in fat to accommodate the dietary needs of individuals who have undergone gastric bypass surgery, and the vegetables are chopped finely to aid in digestion. It's important to consult with a healthcare professional or a dietitian to ensure that this soup fits into your individual dietary plan post-surgery.

The Chicken and Vegetable Soup for gastric bypass patients offers several health benefits:

Nutrient Density: It provides essential nutrients from the chicken and vegetables, including protein, vitamins, and minerals, which are crucial for healing and overall health post-surgery.

Low Fat: The soup is low in fat, which is important for individuals who have undergone gastric bypass surgery to prevent discomfort and aid in digestion.

High Protein: The inclusion of chicken breast ensures that the soup is rich in protein, which is essential for tissue repair, muscle maintenance, and overall health after surgery.

Fiber and Digestive Health: The mixed vegetables provide fiber, aiding in digestion and promoting gut health, which is particularly important after gastric bypass surgery.

Hydration: The broth base of the soup helps with hydration, which is essential for overall health and recovery.

Low Calorie: It's a low-calorie option, helping individuals manage their weight effectively post-surgery.

Lentil Soup

Lentil soup is a nutritious and versatile dish that can be beneficial for individuals who have undergone gastric bypass surgery. This comprehensive guide will explore the nutritional benefits of lentil soup, considerations for gastric bypass patients, and provide a delicious recipe tailored to their dietary needs.

Nutritional Benefits of Lentil Soup:

High Protein Content: Lentils are rich in plant-based protein, making them an excellent choice for gastric bypass patients who need to prioritize protein intake for tissue repair and muscle maintenance.

Low in Fat: Lentils are naturally low in fat, which is beneficial for individuals post-gastric bypass surgery, as high-fat foods can lead to discomfort and digestive issues.

Rich in Fiber: Lentils contain soluble and insoluble fiber, promoting digestive health and regular bowel movements. This can be particularly helpful for gastric bypass patients who may experience changes in bowel habits.

Complex Carbohydrates: Lentils provide complex carbohydrates, which are digested slowly, leading to sustained energy levels and preventing spikes in blood sugar levels.

Nutrient Density: Lentils are packed with essential vitamins and minerals, including iron, folate, potassium, and magnesium, supporting overall health and well-being during the recovery phase after surgery.

Considerations for Gastric Bypass Patients:

Texture: Lentil soup can be blended or pureed to achieve a smoother texture, which may be easier for gastric bypass patients to tolerate, especially in the early stages of recovery.

Portion Size: Gastric bypass patients should be mindful of portion sizes and start with small servings to avoid overeating or discomfort.

Seasoning: Care should be taken with seasoning to avoid excessive use of salt or spices that may trigger digestive issues. Simple seasoning with herbs and spices can enhance flavor without compromising health.

Hydration: Lentil soup provides hydration along with nutrients, which is essential for gastric bypass patients to maintain proper fluid balance and prevent dehydration.

Lentil Soup Recipe for Gastric Bypass Patients:

Ingredients:
1 cup dried lentils, rinsed and drained
4 cups low-sodium vegetable or chicken broth
1 onion, diced
2 carrots, diced
2 celery stalks, diced
2 cloves garlic, minced
1 teaspoon ground cumin

1/2 teaspoon ground turmeric
Salt and pepper to taste
Fresh parsley or cilantro for garnish (optional).

Instructions:
In a large pot, heat a small amount of olive oil over medium heat. Add diced onion, carrots, and celery. Cook until vegetables are softened, about 5 minutes.

To the saucepan, add the ground turmeric, cumin, and chopped garlic. Cook until aromatic, one or two more minutes.

Add rinsed lentils and broth to the pot. Bring to a boil, then reduce heat to low and simmer for 20-25 minutes, or until lentils are tender.
Season with salt and pepper to taste.

Optional: Use an immersion blender to puree the soup to desired consistency.

If preferred, top with chopped cilantro or fresh parsley and serve hot.

Minestrone Soup

Minestrone soup is a hearty and nutritious dish that can be a valuable addition to the diet of individuals who have undergone gastric bypass surgery. This comprehensive guide will explore the nutritional benefits of minestrone soup, considerations for gastric bypass patients, and provide a tailored recipe to meet their dietary needs.

Nutritional Benefits of Minestrone Soup:

Vegetable-Rich: Minestrone soup is typically loaded with a variety of vegetables such as tomatoes, carrots, celery, onions, and spinach. These vegetables provide essential vitamins, minerals, and antioxidants necessary for healing and overall health post-gastric bypass surgery.

Low in Fat: Minestrone soup can be prepared with minimal added fats, making it suitable for individuals who need to limit fat intake after surgery to prevent discomfort and aid digestion.

High Fiber Content: The combination of vegetables, beans, and whole grains in minestrone soup provides a significant amount of dietary fiber. Fiber promotes satiety, aids in digestion, and helps regulate bowel movements, which can be beneficial for gastric bypass patients.

Protein Source: Beans, such as kidney beans, cannellini beans, or chickpeas, are often included in minestrone soup, offering a plant-based source of protein essential for tissue repair and muscle maintenance post-surgery.

Hydration: The broth base of minestrone soup provides hydration, which is crucial for overall health and recovery, particularly after gastric bypass surgery when adequate hydration is essential.

Considerations for Gastric Bypass Patients:

Texture: Depending on individual tolerance levels, the vegetables and beans in minestrone soup can be chopped finely or blended to achieve a smoother texture, which may be easier for gastric bypass patients to tolerate.

Portion Size: Gastric bypass patients should be mindful of portion sizes and start with small servings to prevent overeating or discomfort.

Salt Content: Limiting added salt can help prevent issues such as fluid retention and high blood pressure, which may be more pronounced in individuals who have undergone gastric bypass surgery.

Fat Content: Choose lean protein sources such as beans and limit the use of high-fat ingredients like olive oil or cheese when preparing minestrone soup.

Introduce Gradually: Introduce minestrone soup gradually into the diet post-surgery and monitor tolerance levels to ensure it is well-tolerated.

**Minestrone Soup Recipe for Gastric Bypass
Patients:**

Ingredients:
4 cups low-sodium vegetable or chicken broth
1 can (14 oz) diced tomatoes (no added salt)
1 onion, diced
2 carrots, diced
2 celery stalks, diced
1 zucchini, diced
1 cup cooked beans (such as kidney beans,
cannellini beans, or chickpeas)
1/2 cup whole grain pasta or quinoa (optional)
2 cloves garlic, minced
1 teaspoon dried oregano
1 teaspoon dried basil
Salt and pepper to taste
Fresh parsley for garnish (optional).

Instructions:

In a large pot, combine broth, diced tomatoes, onion, carrots, celery, zucchini, cooked beans, whole grain pasta or quinoa (if using), minced garlic, dried oregano, and dried basil.

Bring the soup to a boil, then reduce the heat and simmer for 20-25 minutes, or until vegetables are tender and flavors have melded together.

Season with salt and pepper to taste.

If desired, top hot dish with fresh parsley.

Turkey Chili

Turkey chili is a savory and filling dish that might provide patients who have had gastric bypass surgery with additional nutrients in their diet. This thorough guide will examine the nutritional advantages of turkey chili, address issues for those who have had gastric bypass surgery, and offer a customized recipe to suit their dietary requirements.

Nutritional Benefits of Turkey Chili:

Lean Protein Source: Turkey is a lean protein source that is lower in fat compared to beef, making it an excellent choice for gastric bypass patients who need to prioritize protein intake for tissue repair and muscle maintenance.

High in Protein: Protein is essential for post-surgery recovery and helps promote satiety, aiding in weight management.

Low in Fat: Turkey chili can be prepared with minimal added fats, making it suitable for individuals who need to limit fat intake after surgery to prevent discomfort and aid digestion.

Fiber-Rich: Beans, vegetables, and tomatoes are common ingredients in turkey chili, providing dietary fiber that promotes digestion, regulates bowel movements, and helps maintain gut health.

Nutrient-Dense: Turkey chili is packed with essential vitamins and minerals from vegetables and spices, including vitamin A, vitamin C, potassium, and iron, supporting overall health and well-being post-gastric bypass surgery.

Considerations for Gastric Bypass Patients:

Texture: Ground turkey and beans in chili may need to be finely chopped or mashed to achieve a smoother texture, which may be easier for gastric bypass patients to tolerate, especially in the early stages of recovery.

Portion Size: Gastric bypass patients should be mindful of portion sizes and start with small servings to prevent overeating or discomfort.

Spice Level: Adjust the level of spices and seasonings according to individual tolerance levels, as some patients may be more sensitive to spicy foods after surgery.

Hydration: Ensure adequate hydration by consuming plenty of fluids alongside turkey chili, as maintaining hydration is crucial for overall health and recovery.

Introduce Gradually: Introduce turkey chili gradually into the diet post-surgery and monitor tolerance levels to ensure it is well-tolerated.

Turkey Chili Recipe for Gastric Bypass Patients:

Ingredients:
Turkey ground, 1 pound, lean
One chopped onion
two minced garlic cloves
One chopped bell pepper and one can (14 oz) of diced tomatoes without salt added
One can (14.2 oz) of washed and drained kidney beans
One can (14.2 oz) of rinsed and drained black beans
One cup of chicken broth with minimal sodium
One tablespoon of powdered chilies
One teaspoon of cumin powder
To taste, add salt and pepper.
Extra toppings at your discretion: sliced avocado, chopped cilantro, and Greek yogurt.

Instructions:
In a large pot, brown ground turkey over medium heat, breaking it apart with a spoon as it cooks.

Add chopped bell pepper, diced onion, and minced garlic to the saucepan. Simmer the veggies for 5 minutes or until they are tender.

Stir in diced tomatoes, drained and rinsed kidney
beans, drained and rinsed black beans, chicken
broth, chili powder, ground cumin, salt, and pepper.

After bringing the chili to a simmer, cook it for
twenty to twenty-five minutes, stirring now and
again, until the flavors have combined and the chili
has thickened.

Adjust seasoning to taste.
Serve hot, garnished with optional toppings such as
chopped cilantro, diced avocado, or a dollop of
Greek yogurt.

CHAPTER SIX

Healthy Desserts

It might be difficult to find dessert selections that are both healthful and appropriate for people who have had gastric bypass surgery. However, it is feasible to enjoy delectable delights that promote healing and general well-being if ingredients and portion proportions are carefully considered. For those who have had gastric bypass surgery, this extensive guide will examine a variety of guilt-free dessert alternatives with an emphasis on portion management, nutrient density, and thoughtful component selection.

Nutritional Considerations for Healthy Desserts:

Portion Control: Gastric bypass patients should be mindful of portion sizes when enjoying desserts to prevent overeating and discomfort. Small, individual servings are often more manageable and allow for better portion control.

Nutrient Density: Choose desserts that are nutrient-dense, meaning they provide essential vitamins, minerals, and other nutrients without excessive calories or added sugars. Option for desserts that incorporate fruits, nuts, seeds, and whole grains for added nutritional value.

Protein-Rich: Including protein in desserts helps promote satiety and supports muscle maintenance and tissue repair post-surgery. Incorporate sources of lean protein such as Greek yogurt, cottage cheese, or protein powder into dessert recipes.

Low in Added Sugars: Minimize the use of added sugars in desserts to avoid spikes in blood sugar levels and promote overall health. Use natural sweeteners such as honey, maple syrup, or fruit purees in moderation.

Fiber Content: Choose desserts that are high in fiber to aid digestion, regulate bowel movements, and promote gut health. Fiber-rich ingredients include fruits, vegetables, whole grains, nuts, and seeds.

Hydration: Consider desserts that incorporate hydrating ingredients such as fruits or yogurt to help maintain proper fluid balance, which is essential for overall health and recovery post-surgery.

Healthy Dessert Options for Gastric Bypass Patients:

Fruit Salad with Greek Yogurt:
Mix together a range of fresh fruits, including citrus fruits, melons, and berries.
For more protein and richness, top with a dollop of Greek yogurt before serving.
For added taste and texture, you can optionally add chopped nuts or a tiny bit of honey.

Baked Apples with Cinnamon and Walnuts:
Apples should be cored, sliced, and put in a baking dish.
After adding some cinnamon, sprinkle chopped walnuts on top.
Bake until the walnuts are gently browned and the apples are soft.
Serve warm, garnished with a handful of crunchy granola or a dollop of Greek yogurt.

Chia Seed Pudding:

Mix chia seeds with milk (such as almond milk or coconut milk) and a natural sweetener like maple syrup or mashed bananas.
The mixture should thicken into the consistency of pudding after being refrigerated for several hours or overnight.
Serve topped with fresh fruit, nuts, or a drizzle of nut butter for added flavor and nutrition.

Protein Smoothie Bowl:
Blend together a combination of frozen fruits, such as berries, bananas, and mangoes, with Greek yogurt or protein powder for added protein.
Pour the smoothie into a bowl and top with additional fruits, nuts, seeds, and a sprinkle of granola or shredded coconut for texture.
Enjoy with a spoon for a refreshing and satisfying dessert option.

Greek Yogurt Popsicles

Greek yogurt popsicles are a delicious and refreshing treat that can be enjoyed by individuals who have undergone gastric bypass surgery. These frozen treats are not only satisfying but also provide essential nutrients such as protein and calcium. This comprehensive guide will explore the benefits of Greek yogurt popsicles for gastric bypass patients, considerations for their dietary needs, and provide a simple recipe to make them at home.

Benefits of Greek Yogurt Popsicles:

High Protein Content: Greek yogurt is an excellent source of protein, which is essential for tissue repair and muscle maintenance post-gastric bypass surgery. Incorporating protein-rich foods like Greek yogurt into desserts helps support recovery and overall health.

Probiotics: Greek yogurt contains beneficial probiotics that promote gut health and digestion, which can be particularly important for individuals who have undergone gastric bypass surgery and may experience digestive issues.

Calcium: Greek yogurt is also rich in calcium, supporting bone health and helping prevent deficiencies that may occur post-surgery due to changes in dietary habits.

Low in Added Sugars: By making Greek yogurt popsicles at home, you can control the amount of added sugars and choose natural sweeteners like honey or fruit purees, making them a healthier option compared to store-bought popsicles.

Hydration: Greek yogurt popsicles provide hydration along with essential nutrients, which is crucial for overall health and recovery, especially in the post-surgery period.

Considerations for Gastric Bypass Patients:

Portion Size: Option for small-sized popsicles to control portion sizes and prevent overeating or discomfort.

Protein Content: Choose Greek yogurt with a high protein content to maximize the nutritional benefits of the popsicles.

Texture: Greek yogurt popsicles have a creamy texture, which may be easier for gastric bypass patients to tolerate compared to icy popsicles. However, individual tolerance levels may vary, so start with small servings and monitor tolerance.

Flavor Variations: Experiment with different flavor combinations using fruits, nuts, seeds, and spices to add variety and excitement to your popsicles while ensuring they meet your dietary needs.

Hydration: Ensure adequate hydration by consuming popsicles alongside water or other hydrating beverages to maintain proper fluid balance post-surgery.

Greek Yogurt Popsicles Recipe for Gastric Bypass Patients:

Ingredients:
2 cups Greek yogurt (low-fat or non-fat)
1-2 tablespoons honey or maple syrup (optional, adjust to taste)
1 teaspoon vanilla extract
1 cup mixed berries (such as strawberries, blueberries, raspberries)
Popsicle molds
Popsicle sticks.

Instructions:
In a mixing bowl, combine Greek yogurt, honey or maple syrup (if using), and vanilla extract. Stir until well combined and smooth.
Wash and chop the mixed berries into small pieces.

Divide the chopped berries evenly among the popsicle molds, filling each mold about halfway. Pour the Greek yogurt mixture over the berries in the molds, filling each mold to the top.

Insert popsicle sticks into each mold.
After the popsicles are fully frozen, place the
popsicle molds in the freezer and freeze for at least
four to six hours.

After the popsicles are frozen, release them from
the molds by briefly running warm water over their
exterior.
Serve the Greek yogurt popsicles immediately and
enjoy!

Berry and Nut Smoothie Bowl

For those who have had gastric bypass surgery, a berry and nut smoothie bowl is a filling and healthy choice. This smoothie bowl is easy on the stomach and full of vital nutrients. It also contains protein, healthy fats, vitamins, and minerals. In-depth discussion of the advantages of berry and nut smoothie bowls for gastric bypass patients, nutritional requirements analysis, and a straightforward recipe for preparing at home are all included in this thorough guide.

Benefits of Berry and Nut Smoothie Bowl:

Nutrient-Dense: A berry and nut smoothie bowl is loaded with nutrients from berries, nuts, seeds, and other wholesome ingredients. It provides essential vitamins, minerals, antioxidants, and phytonutrients that support overall health and well-being post-gastric bypass surgery.

Protein-Rich: Nuts and seeds are excellent sources of plant-based protein, which is essential for tissue repair, muscle maintenance, and overall health post-surgery. Incorporating protein into meals helps promote satiety and aids in weight management.

Healthy Fats: Nuts and seeds are also rich in healthy fats, including omega-3 fatty acids, which are beneficial for heart health and inflammation reduction. Healthy fats help provide sustained energy and promote nutrient absorption.

Fiber Content: Berries, nuts, seeds, and other whole food ingredients in the smoothie bowl provide dietary fiber, which aids digestion, regulates bowel movements, and promotes gut health. Fiber-rich foods are particularly important for gastric bypass patients to prevent constipation and maintain digestive health.

Hydration: Smoothie bowls are typically made with hydrating ingredients such as fruits, vegetables, and liquid bases like almond milk or coconut water, helping individuals maintain proper fluid balance post-surgery.

Considerations for Gastric Bypass Patients:

Texture: Blend the smoothie to achieve a smooth and creamy texture, which may be easier for gastric bypass patients to tolerate compared to chunky textures. Start with small servings and monitor tolerance levels.

Portion Size: Gastric bypass patients should be mindful of portion sizes when enjoying smoothie bowls to prevent overeating or discomfort. Use small bowls and limit the amount of toppings to control portion sizes.

Protein Content: Incorporate protein-rich ingredients like nuts, seeds, Greek yogurt, or protein powder into the smoothie to ensure adequate protein intake post-surgery.

Sugar Content: Limit the use of added sugars in smoothie bowl recipes to avoid spikes in blood sugar levels. Use natural sweeteners like honey, maple syrup, or ripe fruits to sweeten the smoothie.

Toppings: Choose nutritious toppings such as fresh berries, sliced fruits, nuts, seeds, coconut flakes, or granola to add flavor, texture, and additional nutrients to the smoothie bowl.

Berry and Nut Smoothie Bowl Recipe for Gastric Bypass Patients:

Ingredients:
1 cup mixed berries (such as strawberries, blueberries, raspberries)
1 ripe banana
1/2 cup plain Greek yogurt or unsweetened almond milk
1 tablespoon nut butter (such as almond butter or peanut butter)
1 tablespoon chia seeds or ground flaxseeds
Handful of spinach or kale (optional, for added greens)
Toppings: Sliced almonds, walnuts, pumpkin seeds, shredded coconut, fresh berries, sliced banana, granola.

Instructions:

In a blender, combine mixed berries, ripe banana, Greek yogurt or almond milk, nut butter, chia seeds or ground flaxseeds, and spinach or kale (if using).

Blend until creamy and smooth, adding extra liquid as needed to get the right consistency.

Pour the smoothie into a bowl and top with sliced almonds, walnuts, pumpkin seeds, shredded coconut, fresh berries, sliced banana, and granola. Serve immediately and enjoy!

Baked Apples with Cinnamon

Baked apples with cinnamon are a comforting and nutritious dessert option for individuals who have undergone gastric bypass surgery. This simple yet delicious dish is gentle on the stomach and provides essential nutrients, making it suitable for those with altered digestive systems. This comprehensive guide will explore the benefits of baked apples with cinnamon for gastric bypass patients, considerations for their dietary needs, and provide a simple recipe to make them at home.

Benefits of Baked Apples with Cinnamon:

Easy to Digest: Baked apples have a soft and tender texture, making them easy to digest for individuals post-gastric bypass surgery. They are gentle on the stomach and less likely to cause discomfort or digestive issues.

Nutrient-Rich: Apples are a good source of dietary fiber, vitamins, and antioxidants, supporting overall health and well-being post-surgery. Cinnamon adds flavor and may have additional health benefits, such as improving blood sugar control and reducing inflammation.

Low in Added Sugars: Baked apples with cinnamon can be prepared without added sugars, making them a healthier dessert option compared to many store-bought desserts. Natural sweetness from the apples is often sufficient, especially when paired with cinnamon.

Hydration: Apples contain a high water content, contributing to hydration and helping individuals maintain proper fluid balance post-surgery. Adequate hydration is crucial for overall health and recovery.

Portion Control: Baked apples can be portioned according to individual needs, making it easier for gastric bypass patients to control serving sizes and prevent overeating.

Considerations for Gastric Bypass Patients:

Texture: Ensure that the apples are baked until they are soft and tender, making them easier to chew and digest for individuals post-surgery. Monitor tolerance levels and adjust cooking time as needed.

Flavorings: Use minimal added sugars and opt for natural sweeteners like honey or maple syrup, if desired. Cinnamon adds flavor without adding extra calories or sugars, making it a suitable seasoning for gastric bypass patients.

Toppings: Customize baked apples with toppings such as chopped nuts, dried fruits, or a dollop of Greek yogurt for added texture and flavor. Be mindful of portion sizes and choose toppings that align with dietary goals.

Serving Temperature: Serve baked apples warm or at room temperature, as extreme temperatures may be less tolerated by individuals post-gastric bypass surgery. Before serving, let them cool a little.

Variety: Experiment with different types of apples and flavorings to create a variety of baked apple recipes, keeping meals interesting and enjoyable post-surgery.

Baked Apples with Cinnamon Recipe for Gastric Bypass Patients:

Ingredients:
4 medium-sized apples (such as Granny Smith or Honeycrisp)
1 teaspoon ground cinnamon
Optional: 1 tablespoon honey or maple syrup
Optional toppings: Chopped nuts, dried fruits, Greek yogurt.

Instructions:
Preheat the oven to 375°F (190°C).
With the bottoms still on, wash and core the apples.

In a small bowl, mix together cinnamon and honey or maple syrup (if using).

Place the cored apples in a baking dish and fill each cavity with the cinnamon mixture.

Optionally, sprinkle chopped nuts or dried fruits over the top of each apple.

Cover the baking dish with aluminum foil and bake for 25-30 minutes, or until the apples are soft and tender.

Take off the foil and bake for a further five to ten minutes, or until the tops begin to brown a little.

Serve the baked apples warm, optionally topped with a dollop of Greek yogurt or additional toppings of choice.

Dark Chocolate Covered Strawberries

Dark chocolate covered strawberries are a delightful and indulgent treat that can be enjoyed by individuals who have undergone gastric bypass surgery. While being delicious, they also offer potential health benefits due to the antioxidants found in dark chocolate and the vitamins and minerals present in strawberries. This comprehensive guide will explore the benefits of dark chocolate covered strawberries for gastric bypass patients, considerations for their dietary needs, and provide a simple recipe to make them at home.

Benefits of Dark Chocolate Covered Strawberries:

Antioxidant-Rich: Dark chocolate contains antioxidants called flavonoids, which have been associated with various health benefits, including improved heart health and reduced inflammation. Strawberries also contain antioxidants, such as vitamin C, which can help neutralize free radicals in the body.

Heart Health: The flavonoids in dark chocolate may help improve blood flow, lower blood pressure, and reduce the risk of heart disease. Consuming dark chocolate in moderation as part of a balanced diet may contribute to overall heart health for gastric bypass patients.

Nutrient Density: Strawberries are rich in essential vitamins and minerals, including vitamin C, manganese, and folate. Incorporating strawberries into desserts like dark chocolate covered strawberries provides additional nutrients that support overall health and well-being post-surgery.

Portion Control: Dark chocolate covered strawberries can be portioned according to individual needs, making it easier for gastric bypass patients to control serving sizes and prevent overeating. Enjoying them in moderation as part of a balanced diet can satisfy cravings without derailing dietary goals.

Mood Boosting: Dark chocolate contains compounds that may help improve mood and reduce stress by stimulating the release of endorphins and serotonin in the brain. Enjoying a small serving of dark chocolate covered strawberries can provide a mood-boosting treat for gastric bypass patients.

Considerations for Gastric Bypass Patients:

Portion Size: Limit portion sizes of dark chocolate covered strawberries to control calorie intake and prevent discomfort or digestive issues. Enjoying a few strawberries dipped in dark chocolate can satisfy cravings without overindulging.

Dark Chocolate Content: Choose high-quality dark chocolate with a cocoa content of at least 70% to maximize potential health benefits and minimize added sugars. Look for dark chocolate brands with minimal added ingredients and avoid varieties with excessive additives or fillers.

Toppings: Experiment with different toppings to enhance flavor and texture, such as chopped nuts, shredded coconut, or a drizzle of melted white chocolate. Be mindful of portion sizes and choose toppings that align with dietary goals.

Preparation: Wash and dry strawberries thoroughly before dipping them in melted dark chocolate. Ensure that the strawberries are completely dry to prevent the chocolate from seizing or becoming grainy during the dipping process.

Storage: Store dark chocolate covered strawberries in the refrigerator for up to a few days in an airtight container. Enjoy them chilled for a refreshing and satisfying treat.

Dark Chocolate Covered Strawberries Recipe for Gastric Bypass Patients:

Ingredients:
1 cup dark chocolate chips or chopped dark chocolate (at least 70% cocoa content)
One pint of freshly picked strawberries, well cleaned and dried

Optional toppings: Chopped nuts, shredded coconut, melted white chocolate.

Instructions:
Grease a baking sheet or tray with cooking parchment.

In a microwave-safe bowl, melt the dark chocolate in 30-second intervals, stirring between each interval until smooth and fully melted.

Hold each strawberry by the stem and dip it into the melted dark chocolate, coating it halfway or fully as desired.

Allow any excess chocolate to drip off the strawberry, then place it onto the prepared baking sheet.

Optionally, sprinkle toppings such as chopped nuts or shredded coconut over the wet chocolate before it sets.
With the remaining strawberries, repeat the dipping procedure.

If desired, drizzle melted white chocolate over the dipped strawberries for added decoration and flavor.

Place the baking sheet in the refrigerator for about 30 minutes, or until the chocolate has hardened.

Once the chocolate has set, transfer the dark chocolate covered strawberries to an airtight container and store them in the refrigerator until ready to serve.

CHAPTER SEVEN

Beverages

Selecting the appropriate drinks is crucial for people who have had gastric bypass surgery. It's important to pay attention to food intake, proper hydration, and potential digestive problems. This thorough guide will examine appropriate beverage choices for people undergoing gastric bypass surgery, emphasizing nutritional value, hydration, and potential post-surgical difficulties.

Hydration:

Water: Water is the best choice for hydration post-gastric bypass surgery. It is calorie-free, essential for overall health, and helps prevent dehydration.

Herbal Tea: Herbal teas like chamomile, peppermint, or ginger tea are soothing and can aid digestion. Option for caffeine-free varieties to avoid potential stomach irritation.

Infused Water: Add flavor to water with slices of citrus fruits, cucumber, or fresh herbs like mint or basil for a refreshing twist without added sugars.

Nutritional Considerations:

Protein Shakes: Protein shakes can help meet daily protein needs post-surgery. Choose low-sugar, high-protein options and dilute them with water to prevent overwhelming the stomach.

Low-Fat Milk: Skim or low-fat milk provides protein, calcium, and vitamins without excess fat. Lactose-free options may be easier to digest for some patients.

Vegetable Juice: Homemade vegetable juices can be nutrient-rich and hydrating. Blend vegetables like spinach, kale, carrots, and cucumbers for a refreshing beverage high in vitamins and minerals.

Bone Broth: Bone broth is rich in protein, collagen, and minerals, aiding in healing and supporting gut health. Choose low-sodium varieties or make your own broth at home.

Challenges and Considerations:

Carbonated Beverages: Carbonated beverages can cause discomfort or bloating post-surgery. Avoid carbonated drinks, including soda and sparkling water, especially in the early stages of recovery.

High-Sugar Beverages: Sugary drinks like soda, fruit juices, and sweetened beverages should be limited or avoided to prevent dumping syndrome, blood sugar spikes, and weight gain.

Alcohol: Alcohol should be consumed sparingly, if at all, post-gastric bypass surgery. It can be more potent and may lead to increased intoxication and nutrient malabsorption.

Caffeine: Caffeinated beverages like coffee, tea, and energy drinks can irritate the stomach lining and increase stomach acid production. Limit caffeine intake and opt for decaffeinated versions or herbal teas.

Tips for Beverage Consumption:

Sip slowly: Take small sips of beverages throughout the day to prevent overloading the stomach and minimize discomfort.

Track intake: Keep track of fluid intake to ensure adequate hydration, especially in the early stages of recovery when fluid needs may be higher.

Avoid straws: Drinking through a straw can introduce excess air into the stomach, leading to bloating or discomfort. Instead, sip straight from a glass or cup.

Choose nutrient-dense options: Option for beverages that provide essential nutrients to support recovery and overall health post-surgery.

Protein Shakes and Smoothies

Smoothies and protein drinks are great additions to the diet for those who have had gastric bypass surgery. These drinks offer vital nutrients in a handy and easily digested form, such as protein, vitamins, and minerals. This thorough guide will examine the advantages of protein shakes and smoothies for those after gastric bypass surgery, take into account their nutritional requirements, and offer advice on how to make wholesome and filling drinks at home.

Benefits of Protein Shakes and Smoothies:

Protein-Rich: Protein shakes and smoothies are an excellent way to increase protein intake post-gastric bypass surgery, supporting tissue repair, muscle maintenance, and overall health.

Nutrient-Dense: By incorporating ingredients like fruits, vegetables, dairy or plant-based milk, and protein sources such as protein powder or Greek yogurt, protein shakes and smoothies provide essential vitamins, minerals, and antioxidants.

Hydration: Adding liquid components like water, milk, or coconut water to protein shakes and smoothies helps maintain proper hydration, which is crucial for overall health and recovery post-surgery.

Easily Digestible: Blending ingredients into a smooth, liquid form makes protein shakes and smoothies easier to digest, reducing the risk of discomfort or digestive issues commonly experienced after gastric bypass surgery.

Convenient: Protein shakes and smoothies are quick and convenient meal or snack options for gastric bypass patients, especially during the initial stages of recovery when appetite and eating capacity may be limited.

Considerations for Gastric Bypass Patients:

Protein Content: Choose protein sources with high bioavailability and minimal added sugars, such as whey protein isolate or plant-based protein powders. Aim for at least 20-30 grams of protein per serving to support post-surgery nutritional needs.

Liquid Base: Use low-fat dairy milk, unsweetened almond milk, coconut water, or water as the liquid base for protein shakes and smoothies. Avoid high-sugar fruit juices or sweetened beverages that can contribute to dumping syndrome or weight gain.

Fruit Selection: Option for low-sugar fruits like berries, citrus fruits, and apples in protein shakes and smoothies. Limit or avoid high-sugar fruits like bananas, mangoes, and pineapple, which can spike blood sugar levels.

Fiber Content: Incorporate fiber-rich ingredients like spinach, kale, chia seeds, or ground flaxseeds to promote digestion, regulate bowel movements, and support gut health post-surgery.

Texture: Blend ingredients until smooth and creamy to achieve a texture that is easily tolerated by gastric bypass patients. Avoid adding chunks or large pieces of ingredients that may be difficult to digest.

Tips for Creating Protein Shakes and Smoothies:

Balance Macronutrients: Include a balance of protein, carbohydrates, and healthy fats in protein shakes and smoothies to support energy levels, satiety, and overall nutrition.

Experiment with Flavors: Add natural flavorings like vanilla extract, cinnamon, or cocoa powder to enhance the taste of protein shakes and smoothies without adding extra calories or sugars.

Pre-Portion Ingredients: Pre-portion ingredients like fruits, vegetables, and protein powder into individual servings to streamline preparation and ensure consistent nutrient content.

Drink Mindfully: Sip protein shakes and smoothies slowly and mindfully to prevent overconsumption and allow time for the stomach to adjust to liquid intake post-surgery.

Customize to Preferences: Customize protein shakes and smoothies to suit individual taste preferences and dietary restrictions, experimenting with different ingredients and flavor combinations.

Protein shakes and smoothies offer critical nutrients in a digestible and pleasant form, making them a healthy and practical choice for individuals undergoing gastric bypass surgery. Following surgery, people may enhance their recuperation and general well-being by consuming foods high in nutrients, using thoughtful cooking methods, and using high-quality protein sources. Always seek the advice of a medical expert before making any dietary changes in light of your unique demands and medical background.

Herbal Teas

Herbal teas are soothing and hydrating beverages that can be beneficial for individuals who have undergone gastric bypass surgery. These teas offer various flavors and potential health benefits without the addition of caffeine or excessive sugars. This comprehensive guide will explore the benefits of herbal teas for gastric bypass patients, considerations for their dietary needs, and provide information on different types of herbal teas suitable for post-surgery consumption.

Benefits of Herbal Teas:

Hydration: Herbal teas provide hydration, which is essential for overall health and recovery post-gastric bypass surgery. Staying hydrated helps prevent dehydration, supports digestion, and aids in nutrient absorption.

Soothing Properties: Many herbal teas have soothing properties that can help alleviate digestive discomfort, bloating, or nausea commonly experienced after gastric bypass surgery. Ingredients like ginger, peppermint, and chamomile are known for their calming effects on the stomach.

Caffeine-Free: Herbal teas are naturally caffeine-free, making them suitable for individuals who need to limit caffeine intake post-surgery. Avoiding caffeine helps prevent potential stomach irritation and promotes better sleep quality.

Antioxidants: Some herbal teas contain antioxidants that can help reduce inflammation, support immune function, and protect against oxidative stress. Ingredients like hibiscus, rooibos, and green tea provide beneficial antioxidants without the stimulating effects of caffeine.

Variety of Flavors: Herbal teas come in a wide range of flavors and blends, allowing individuals post-surgery to enjoy a variety of tastes without the need for added sugars or artificial flavorings.

Considerations for Gastric Bypass Patients:

Avoiding Irritants: Choose herbal teas that are gentle on the stomach and avoid ingredients that may irritate the digestive system, such as black tea, which contains tannins that can cause stomach upset.

Sipping Mindfully: Sip herbal teas slowly and mindfully to prevent overconsumption and allow the stomach to adjust to liquid intake post-surgery. Avoid drinking large volumes of liquids in a short period, which can lead to discomfort or bloating.

Monitoring Ingredients: Read labels carefully to ensure herbal teas do not contain added sugars, artificial sweeteners, or other ingredients that may be problematic post-surgery. Option for natural, pure herbal teas without additives or preservatives.

Experimenting with Blends: Experiment with different herbal tea blends and flavors to find ones that are soothing, enjoyable, and well-tolerated post-surgery. Customize teas with ingredients like fresh ginger, lemon, or honey for added flavor and benefits.

Temperature: Allow herbal teas to cool slightly before drinking to avoid potential irritation to the stomach lining. Drinking teas at a moderate temperature can help prevent discomfort or burning sensations.

Types of Herbal Teas Suitable for Gastric Bypass Patients:

Peppermint Tea: Peppermint tea is known for its soothing properties and can help relieve digestive discomfort, bloating, and nausea post-surgery.

Ginger Tea: Ginger tea has anti-inflammatory and digestive benefits, making it ideal for gastric bypass patients experiencing digestive issues or nausea.

Chamomile Tea: Chamomile tea is calming and may help promote relaxation, reduce stress, and aid digestion, making it a soothing option post-surgery.

Rooibos Tea: Rooibos tea is caffeine-free and rich in antioxidants, offering potential health benefits without the stimulating effects of caffeine.

Herbal Blends: Explore herbal tea blends that combine ingredients like chamomile, lavender, and lemon balm for a calming and aromatic experience.

Infused Water

Infused water is a flavorful and refreshing beverage option for individuals who have undergone gastric bypass surgery. It provides hydration while offering subtle hints of natural flavors from fruits, vegetables, and herbs. This comprehensive guide will explore the benefits of infused water for gastric bypass patients, considerations for their dietary needs, and provide tips for creating delicious infused water combinations at home.

Benefits of Infused Water:

Hydration: Staying hydrated is essential for gastric bypass patients to support overall health, aid digestion, and promote recovery. Infused water provides a flavorful alternative to plain water, making it easier to meet daily fluid intake goals.

Natural Flavor: Infused water adds natural flavor to water without the need for added sugars, artificial sweeteners, or flavorings. The subtle taste of fruits, vegetables, and herbs enhances the drinking experience and encourages hydration.

Low-Calorie: Infused water is low in calories, making it suitable for individuals post-surgery who need to manage calorie intake and maintain weight loss. It provides a refreshing beverage option without contributing excess calories or sugars.

Antioxidants and Nutrients: Fruits, vegetables, and herbs used in infused water may release antioxidants, vitamins, and minerals into the water, offering potential health benefits. Ingredients like citrus fruits, berries, cucumber, and mint provide vitamins and antioxidants that support overall well-being.

Variety and Customization: Infused water allows for endless flavor combinations and customization options. Individuals post-surgery can experiment with different fruits, vegetables, and herbs to create personalized infused water blends that suit their taste preferences.

Considerations for Gastric Bypass Patients:

Gentle Flavors: Choose fruits, vegetables, and herbs with gentle flavors that are well-tolerated post-surgery. Avoid ingredients that may cause digestive discomfort or irritation, such as spicy peppers or strong herbs.

Monitor Intake: Keep track of infused water intake to ensure adequate hydration throughout the day. Sip infused water slowly and consistently to prevent dehydration and support overall health.

Avoid Added Sugars: Avoid adding sweeteners like sugar, honey, or syrup to infused water, as they can contribute unnecessary calories and may lead to dumping syndrome or blood sugar spikes.

Temperature: Enjoy infused water at a moderate temperature to prevent discomfort or irritation to the stomach lining. Avoid consuming extremely cold or hot beverages, especially in the early stages of recovery.

Fresh Ingredients: Use fresh, high-quality ingredients to infuse water for the best flavor and nutritional value. Wash fruits, vegetables, and herbs thoroughly before adding them to water to remove any dirt or pesticides.

Tips for Creating Infused Water:

Slice or Muddle Ingredients: Slice fruits and vegetables thinly or muddle them gently to release their natural flavors into the water more effectively.

Combine Flavors: Experiment with different combinations of fruits, vegetables, and herbs to create unique and refreshing infused water blends. Some popular combinations include cucumber and mint, lemon and basil, or strawberry and lime.

Let it Infuse: Allow infused water to sit for at least 1-2 hours, or overnight in the refrigerator, to allow the flavors to fully infuse into the water. The longer it sits, the more flavorful the infused water will become.

Refresh Ingredients: Refresh infused water by adding fresh ingredients or changing the flavor combinations regularly. Replace used ingredients every 24-48 hours for optimal flavor and freshness.

Customize to Taste: Adjust the intensity of flavor by adding more or fewer ingredients according to personal taste preferences. Start with a small amount of ingredients and adjust as needed to achieve the desired flavor.

CHAPTER EIGHT

Special Occasion and Holiday Recipes

Special occasions and holidays are times for celebration and gathering with loved ones, often centered around food. For individuals who have undergone gastric bypass surgery, navigating these events while adhering to dietary guidelines can be challenging. However, with thoughtful planning and creative recipes, it's possible to enjoy delicious and festive meals without compromising post-surgery health goals. This comprehensive guide will explore special occasion and holiday recipes tailored for gastric bypass patients, focusing on flavorful, nutrient-dense dishes that are gentle on the stomach and promote overall well-being.

Appetizers:

Caprese Skewers: Cherry tomatoes, mozzarella balls, and fresh basil leaves should all be threaded onto skewers. Add a balsamic glaze drizzle for a tasty and eye-catching appetizer.

Cucumber Avocado Rolls: Spread mashed avocado on cucumber slices and roll them up. Secure with toothpicks and garnish with a sprinkle of black sesame seeds for an elegant appetizer option.

Main Courses:

Herb-Roasted Turkey Breast: Roast a boneless turkey breast seasoned with a blend of herbs like rosemary, thyme, and sage. Serve with homemade cranberry sauce and steamed green beans for a classic holiday meal.

Lemon Garlic Shrimp Skewers: Marinate shrimp in a mixture of lemon juice, garlic, and olive oil, then skewer and grill until cooked through. Serve with a side of roasted vegetables for a light and flavorful main course.

Side Dishes:

Cauliflower Mash: Steam cauliflower florets until tender, then mash with a potato masher or blend until smooth. Season with garlic powder, salt, and pepper for a low-carb alternative to mashed potatoes.

Roasted Brussels Sprouts with Bacon: Toss halved Brussels sprouts with olive oil, salt, and pepper, then roast until caramelized. Sprinkle cooked bacon pieces over the top before serving for added flavor.

Desserts:

Mini Cheesecake Bites: Prepare individual cheesecake bites using a mixture of Greek yogurt, cream cheese, and sweetener of choice. Top with fresh berries and a drizzle of sugar-free chocolate sauce for a decadent treat.

Pumpkin Spice Protein Pudding: Mix pumpkin puree with protein powder, pumpkin pie spice, and a splash of almond milk until smooth. Chill in the refrigerator until set, then top with a dollop of whipped cream and a sprinkle of cinnamon.

Beverages:

Sparkling Berry Mocktail: Combine sparkling water with mixed berry puree and a squeeze of fresh lime juice. Serve over ice with a garnish of mint leaves for a refreshing and festive drink.

Cinnamon Apple Spice Tea: Brew cinnamon apple herbal tea and serve warm with a cinnamon stick for stirring. Add a slice of fresh apple for garnish and extra flavor.

Considerations for Gastric Bypass Patients:

Portion Control: Serve smaller portion sizes to prevent overeating and discomfort post-surgery.
Protein Focus: Incorporate protein-rich ingredients into each meal to support recovery and maintain muscle mass.

Hydration: Encourage guests to stay hydrated by offering a variety of non-alcoholic beverages throughout the event.
Mindful Eating: Encourage mindful eating practices, such as chewing slowly and savoring each bite, to prevent overconsumption and aid digestion.

Thanksgiving Turkey with Low-Carb Stuffing

Thanksgiving is a time for gathering with loved ones and enjoying a hearty feast, but for individuals who have undergone gastric bypass surgery, traditional holiday meals can present challenges. However, with some creative adaptations, it's possible to create a delicious and satisfying Thanksgiving turkey with low-carb stuffing that is gentle on the stomach and aligns with post-surgery dietary guidelines. This comprehensive guide will explore how to prepare a Thanksgiving turkey with low-carb stuffing, considerations for gastric bypass patients, and tips for making the holiday meal enjoyable and memorable.

Ingredients:

Turkey: Choose a bone-in turkey breast or whole turkey, depending on the size of your gathering and preference. Option for lean cuts of turkey to minimize fat content.

Low-Carb Stuffing Ingredients:

Cauliflower Rice: Substitute traditional bread stuffing with cauliflower rice for a low-carb alternative.
Vegetables: Include chopped onions, celery, mushrooms, and bell peppers for flavor and texture.
Herbs and Seasonings: Use a blend of fresh herbs like sage, thyme, and rosemary, along with salt, pepper, and garlic powder for seasoning.
Optional Additions: Add diced cooked turkey sausage or chopped nuts for extra protein and flavor.

Instructions:

Preparing the Turkey:
Thaw the turkey according to package instructions, if frozen. Remove giblets and rinse the turkey under cold water, then pat dry with paper towels.
Preheat the oven to the appropriate temperature (usually 325°F to 350°F).
Season the turkey with salt, pepper, and your choice of herbs and seasonings, both inside and out. Place the turkey breast-side up in a roasting pan.

Making the Low-Carb Stuffing:

In a large skillet, sauté chopped onions, celery, mushrooms, and bell peppers in olive oil until softened.

Add cauliflower rice to the skillet and continue cooking until tender.

Season the mixture with herbs, salt, pepper, and garlic powder to taste. Stir in any optional additions, such as cooked turkey sausage or chopped nuts.

Remove the skillet from heat and let the stuffing mixture cool slightly before using it to stuff the turkey.

Stuffing the Turkey:

Spoon the low-carb stuffing mixture into the cavity of the turkey, packing it loosely to allow for even cooking.

If there is leftover stuffing, place it in a separate baking dish and bake it alongside the turkey.

Roasting the Turkey:

Loosely place foil over the turkey and bake it in the preheated oven in accordance with the weight and cooking guidelines that came with it.

In order to allow the skin of the turkey to brown, remove the foil during the last hour of cooking.

Make sure the turkey achieves the proper internal
temperature (165°F for poultry) by using a meat
thermometer.

Considerations for Gastric Bypass Patients:

Portion Control: Serve smaller portions of turkey
and stuffing to prevent overeating and discomfort
post-surgery.

Protein Focus: Prioritize consuming the
protein-rich turkey meat over the stuffing to meet
nutritional needs and support recovery.

Low-Carb Options: Choose low-carb side dishes
and desserts to complement the turkey, such as
roasted vegetables, salad, and sugar-free cranberry
sauce.

Hydration: Encourage guests to stay hydrated by
offering water or other non-alcoholic beverages
throughout the meal.

Christmas Roast Beef with Vegetable Medley

celebration and indulgence, it's crucial for those who have had gastric bypass surgery to make conscious decisions that support their health objectives. An excellent and filling dinner choice that is rich in nutrients, flavorful, and easy on the stomach is a Christmas roast beef with vegetable medley. This extensive manual will go over how to make a vegetable medley and roast beef for Christmas, as well as what to know about gastric bypass patients and how to make the holiday feast fun and festive without going overboard with diet restrictions.

Ingredients:

Roast Beef:

Lean Beef Roast: Choose a lean cut of beef, such as sirloin, tenderloin, or eye of round, to minimize fat content.

Herbs and Spices: Use a blend of herbs and spices for seasoning, such as rosemary, thyme, garlic powder, salt, and pepper.
Olive Oil: Use olive oil for coating the beef roast and enhancing flavor.

Vegetable Medley:

Assorted Vegetables: Choose a variety of colorful vegetables, such as carrots, broccoli, cauliflower, bell peppers, zucchini, and Brussels sprouts.
Olive Oil: Use olive oil for roasting the vegetables and adding richness.
Herbs and Seasonings: Season the vegetables with herbs like thyme, oregano, or parsley, along with salt and pepper for flavor.

Instructions:

Preparing the Roast Beef:
Preheat the oven to the appropriate temperature (usually 325°F to 350°F).
Season the beef roast with herbs, spices, salt, and pepper, rubbing them evenly over the surface of the meat.

Slightly warm up a skillet on medium-high heat and drizzle with olive oil. Browning occurs as the beef roast is seared on both sides.

Transfer the seared beef roast to a roasting pan and roast it in the preheated oven until it reaches the desired level of doneness, using a meat thermometer to gauge internal temperature.

Roasting the Vegetable Medley:
While the beef roast is cooking, prepare the vegetable medley.

Wash and chop the assorted vegetables into bite-sized pieces, ensuring they are uniform in size for even cooking.

Toss the vegetables with olive oil, herbs, salt, and pepper until evenly coated.

Spread the seasoned vegetables in a single layer on a baking sheet and roast them in the oven alongside the beef roast until tender and caramelized, stirring occasionally for even cooking.

Serving:
Once the beef roast and vegetable medley are cooked to perfection, remove them from the oven and let them rest for a few minutes before slicing and serving.
Arrange slices of roast beef on a platter alongside the roasted vegetable medley for a colorful and festive presentation.
Garnish with fresh herbs or a drizzle of olive oil, if desired, before serving.

Considerations for Gastric Bypass Patients:

Portion Control: Serve smaller portions of roast beef and vegetables to prevent overeating and discomfort post-surgery.
Protein Focus: Prioritize consuming the protein-rich beef roast to meet nutritional needs and support recovery.

Vegetable Variety: Choose a variety of colorful vegetables for the medley to ensure a diverse range of nutrients and flavors.

Seasoning Options: Experiment with different herbs and spices to customize the flavor profile of both the roast beef and vegetable medley.

Hydration: Encourage guests to stay hydrated by offering water or other non-alcoholic beverages throughout the meal.

Fourth of July Grilled Shrimp Skewers

Fourth of July celebrations often involve outdoor gatherings and delicious grilled foods, but for individuals who have undergone gastric bypass surgery, it's essential to choose options that are gentle on the stomach and align with post-surgery dietary guidelines. Grilled shrimp skewers offer a flavorful and protein-rich option that is easy to digest and perfect for summer festivities. This comprehensive guide will explore how to prepare Fourth of July grilled shrimp skewers, considerations for gastric bypass patients, and tips for making the holiday meal enjoyable and satisfying while maintaining dietary restrictions.

Ingredients:

Shrimp:

Large Shrimp: Choose large, peeled, and deveined shrimp for convenience and ease of preparation.
Olive Oil: Use olive oil for marinating the shrimp and preventing sticking on the grill.

Lemon Juice: Freshly squeezed lemon juice adds brightness and flavor to the shrimp marinade.
Garlic: Minced garlic enhances the flavor of the shrimp marinade.
Seasonings: Use a blend of seasonings such as paprika, cumin, salt, and pepper for added flavor.
Vegetables (Optional):

Assorted Vegetables: Choose vegetables like cherry tomatoes, bell peppers, zucchini, and onions for threading onto the skewers alongside the shrimp.
Olive Oil: Use olive oil for coating the vegetables and enhancing flavor.
Seasonings: Season the vegetables with salt, pepper, and herbs like oregano or thyme for extra flavor.

Skewers:

Skewers: Use metal or wooden skewers for threading the shrimp and vegetables. If using wooden skewers, soak them in water for at least 30 minutes before grilling to prevent burning.

Instructions:

Preparing the Shrimp:
In a bowl, combine the shrimp with olive oil, lemon
juice, minced garlic, and seasonings. Toss to coat
the shrimp evenly in the marinade.
Cover the bowl and refrigerate the shrimp for at
least 30 minutes to allow the flavors to meld.

Preparing the Vegetables (Optional):
If including vegetables on the skewers, wash and
chop them into bite-sized pieces.
In a separate bowl, toss the vegetables with olive
oil, seasonings, and herbs until evenly coated.

Assembling the Skewers:
Preheat the grill to medium-high heat.
Thread the marinated shrimp and optional
vegetables onto the skewers, alternating between
shrimp and vegetables for colorful and flavorful
skewers.

Grilling the Skewers:
Place the assembled skewers on the preheated grill and cook for 2-3 minutes per side, or until the shrimp are pink and opaque.
Flip the skewers halfway through cooking to ensure even grilling on both sides.
Be careful not to overcook the shrimp, as they can become tough and rubbery.

Serving:
Once the shrimp skewers are cooked through, remove them from the grill and transfer them to a serving platter.
Garnish with fresh herbs or a squeeze of lemon juice before serving for added freshness and flavor.

Considerations for Gastric Bypass Patients:

Portion Control: Serve smaller portions of shrimp skewers to prevent overeating and discomfort post-surgery.
Protein Focus: Prioritize consuming the protein-rich shrimp to meet nutritional needs and support recovery.

Vegetable Inclusion: Include a variety of colorful vegetables on the skewers for added nutrients and fiber, but be mindful of portion sizes.

Seasoning Options: Customize the seasonings to suit individual taste preferences and dietary restrictions, avoiding excess salt or spicy seasonings if sensitive.

Hydration: Encourage guests to stay hydrated by offering water or other non-alcoholic beverages throughout the meal.

Birthday Celebration Cake Options

Birthdays are special occasions to celebrate with loved ones, and having undergone gastric bypass surgery doesn't mean missing out on enjoying a delicious cake. However, it's essential to choose cake options that are gentle on the stomach, lower in sugar and fat, and still provide a delightful treat for the celebration. This comprehensive guide will explore various birthday celebration cake options tailored for gastric bypass patients, considerations for dietary restrictions, and tips for making the birthday celebration memorable and enjoyable while maintaining health goals.

Low-Sugar Angel Food Cake:

Ingredients:

Egg Whites: Use egg whites as the base for the cake batter.
Sugar Substitute: Substitute traditional sugar with a sugar substitute like stevia or erythritol.

Flour: Use cake flour or a combination of flour and cornstarch for a lighter texture.

Vanilla Extract: Add vanilla extract for flavor.
Cream of Tartar: Use cream of tartar to stabilize the egg whites and create a fluffy texture.

Instructions:
Set up a tube pan and preheat the oven.
Cream of tartar is added to egg whites and beaten until firm peaks form.
While beating, gradually add the sugar replacement and vanilla essence.
Add the flour mixture and gently fold until well blended.
After pouring the batter onto the ready pan, bake it until it turns golden brown.
Before serving, let the cake cool fully.

Sugar-Free Cheesecake:

Ingredients:

Cream Cheese: Use reduced-fat cream cheese or Greek yogurt for a lighter version.
Sugar Substitute: Substitute sugar with a sugar-free sweetener.

Eggs: Use eggs to bind the cheesecake filling.

Almond Flour Crust (optional): Make a crust using almond flour, butter, and a sugar substitute.

Instructions:
Warm up the oven and get a springform pan ready. Cream cheese should be smoothed out before adding the sugar replacement and mixing thoroughly.
One egg at a time, adding and thoroughly mixing after each addition.
Pour the filling into the prepared crust, if using, or directly into the pan.
Bake the cheesecake until set and slightly golden. Chill the cheesecake in the refrigerator before serving.

Protein-Packed Flourless Chocolate Cake:

Ingredients:

Black Beans: Use canned black beans as the base for the cake.
Cocoa Powder: Add cocoa powder for a rich chocolate flavor.
Eggs: Use eggs to bind the cake together.
Sugar Substitute: Use a sugar substitute to sweeten the cake.
Vanilla Extract: Add vanilla extract for flavor.

Instructions:
Assemble a cake pan and preheat the oven.
After the black beans have been rinsed and drained, mix them with cocoa powder until smooth.
Blend together the eggs, sugar substitute, and vanilla extract in the blender until well blended.
Fill the pan with the batter, then bake it until it solidifies.

Chill the cake completely before cutting.

Considerations for Gastric Bypass Patients:

Portion Control: Serve smaller slices of cake to prevent overeating and discomfort post-surgery.
Sugar Substitutes: Choose sugar substitutes that are safe for consumption post-surgery and do not cause digestive issues.
Protein Focus: Incorporate protein-rich ingredients like Greek yogurt or black beans into the cake for added nutritional benefits.
Texture and Moisture: Option for cake options that are moist and tender to avoid dryness and difficulty swallowing.
Hydration: Drink water or other non-caloric beverages alongside cake consumption to aid digestion and prevent dehydration.

CHAPTER NINE

Meal Prep Tips and Ideas

Meal prep is a valuable tool for individuals who have undergone gastric bypass surgery, as it allows for convenient, portion-controlled meals that align with post-surgery dietary guidelines. Effective meal prep can help ensure balanced nutrition, promote weight management, and simplify mealtime, making it easier to adhere to dietary restrictions and support long-term success. This comprehensive guide will explore meal prep tips and ideas specifically tailored for gastric bypass patients, including considerations for portion control, nutrient balance, and flavor variety.

Meal Prep Tips:

Plan Ahead: Take time to plan your meals for the week, including breakfast, lunch, dinner, and snacks. Consider your nutritional needs, dietary preferences, and any special occasions or events that may influence meal choices.

Choose Nutrient-Dense Foods: Focus on incorporating lean protein sources, non-starchy vegetables, healthy fats, and whole grains into your meal prep. Prioritize foods that provide essential nutrients while being gentle on the stomach and promoting satiety.

Portion Control: Use portion control tools such as measuring cups, food scales, or portioned containers to ensure proper serving sizes. Gastric bypass patients have smaller stomach capacities, so portion control is crucial to prevent overeating and discomfort.

Cook in Batches: Save time and energy by cooking large batches of protein, grains, and vegetables that can be portioned and stored for multiple meals throughout the week. Choose versatile ingredients that can be used in various recipes to maximize efficiency.

Incorporate Variety: Keep meals interesting and enjoyable by incorporating a variety of flavors, textures, and cuisines into your meal prep. Experiment with different recipes, spices, and cooking methods to prevent boredom and promote adherence to dietary guidelines.

Include Ready-to-Eat Options: Prepare grab-and-go snacks and meals that require minimal preparation, such as pre-cut vegetables with hummus, Greek yogurt with fruit, or boiled eggs. Having convenient options readily available can help prevent unhealthy food choices when hunger strikes.

Practice Safe Food Handling: Follow proper food safety practices when preparing, cooking, and storing meals to prevent foodborne illness. Wash hands frequently, store perishable foods in the refrigerator or freezer promptly, and reheat leftovers to the proper temperature before consuming.

Meal Prep Ideas:

Protein-Based Meals:
quinoa, grilled chicken breast, and roasted veggies.
Brown rice and steamed broccoli paired with baked
salmon.
Marinara sauce-topped turkey meatballs
accompanied with zucchini noodles.

Vegetarian Options:
Lentil and vegetable stew served with a side of
mixed greens.
Tofu stir-fry with bell peppers, snap peas, and
brown rice.
Cucumber, cherry tomatoes, feta cheese, and
chickpea salad.

Breakfast Ideas:
Crustless quiche cups with spinach, mushrooms,
and low-fat cheese.
Greek yogurt parfait with granola and fresh berries.

Egg muffins with turkey sausage and diced vegetables.

Snack Options:
Cottage cheese with sliced fruit and almonds.
Whole grain crackers and carrot sticks go well with hummus.
Protein smoothie made with Greek yogurt, spinach, and frozen berries.

Considerations for Gastric Bypass Patients:

Focus on Protein: Prioritize protein-rich foods to support muscle maintenance, promote satiety, and aid in recovery post-surgery.

Choose Nutrient-Dense Foods: Select foods that provide essential nutrients without excess calories, sugars, or fats to support overall health and well-being.

Monitor Hydration: Stay hydrated throughout the day by drinking water or other calorie-free beverages between meals to prevent dehydration and promote optimal digestion.

Listen to Your Body: Pay attention to hunger and fullness cues, and eat slowly to prevent discomfort or dumping syndrome. Even if there is food left on your plate, you should stop eating when you are full.

In summary, meal preparation can help gastric bypass patients adhere to dietary recommendations, encourage nutritional balance, and streamline mealtimes. Following surgery, people may support their health and well-being by planning ahead, selecting nutrient-dense foods, controlling portion sizes, and adding diversity to meal prep. Both of these strategies will help them enjoy tasty and fulfilling meals. Try out various meal combinations, ingredients, and recipes to see what suits your needs and tastes the best. For individualized dietary advice based on your unique medical history and nutritional needs, always speak with a medical expert or registered dietitian.

Batch Cooking for Convenience

Batch cooking is a practical and time-saving approach to meal preparation that can greatly benefit individuals who have undergone gastric bypass surgery. By cooking larger quantities of food at once and portioning it into meals for the week, batch cooking ensures that gastric bypass patients have convenient, portion-controlled options readily available, reducing the temptation to make less healthy choices when time is limited.

Benefits of Batch Cooking for Gastric Bypass Patients:

Time Efficiency: Batch cooking allows individuals to prepare multiple meals at once, saving time on meal prep throughout the week. This is especially beneficial for those with busy schedules or limited time for cooking.

Portion Control: Batch cooking enables portion control by dividing meals into pre-portioned servings, ensuring that gastric bypass patients consume appropriate portion sizes to prevent overeating and promote weight management.

Consistency: Batch cooking promotes consistency in meal choices, making it easier to adhere to dietary guidelines and avoid impulse eating or unhealthy snacking.

Cost Savings: Cooking in bulk can be more cost-effective than preparing individual meals, as ingredients can be purchased in larger quantities and used across multiple dishes.

Variety: Batch cooking allows for versatility in meal options by preparing different dishes in advance, providing variety throughout the week without the need for extensive daily meal preparation.

Tips for Batch Cooking for Gastric Bypass Patients:

Plan Your Meals: Start by planning your meals for the week, taking into account your nutritional needs, dietary preferences, and any special occasions or events.

Pick Versatile items: To increase productivity and reduce waste, use items that may be utilized in a variety of dishes. Lean meats, nutritious grains, and an assortment of veggies are a few examples.

Invest in Storage Containers: Purchase a selection of portioned storage containers in various sizes to accommodate different meal sizes and prevent overfilling.

Use Time-Saving Cooking Methods: Utilize time-saving cooking methods such as roasting, grilling, or slow cooking to prepare large batches of food with minimal hands-on time.

Label and Date Containers: Label each container with the name of the dish and the date it was prepared to ensure freshness and prevent confusion.

Store Properly: Store batch-cooked meals in the refrigerator or freezer according to recommended storage guidelines to maintain freshness and food safety.

Rotate Your Meals: Rotate your batch-cooked meals throughout the week to ensure variety and prevent monotony.

Meal Ideas Suitable for Batch Cooking:

Lean Protein Options:
Grilled chicken breasts
Baked salmon filets
Turkey meatballs

Lentil stew.

Whole Grain Dishes:
Quinoa salad
Brown rice pilaf
Whole wheat pasta with marinara sauce.

Vegetable-Based Recipes:
Roasted mixed vegetables
Stir-fried vegetables with tofu
Vegetable soup or stew.

Breakfast Options:
Egg muffins with spinach and feta cheese
Overnight oats with mixed berries
Greek yogurt parfaits with granola and fruit.

Considerations for Gastric Bypass Patients:

Focus on Protein: Prioritize protein-rich ingredients in batch-cooked meals to support muscle maintenance and promote satiety.

Portion Control: Use portioned containers to divide batch-cooked meals into appropriate serving sizes, taking into account individual dietary needs and post-surgery restrictions.

Monitor Hydration: Drink water or other calorie-free beverages between meals to stay hydrated and support optimal digestion.

Listen to Your Body: Pay attention to hunger and fullness cues, and eat slowly to prevent discomfort or dumping syndrome. Even if there is food left on your plate, you should stop eating when you are full.

Freezing and Reheating Guidelines

Freezing and reheating meals can be a convenient and time-saving strategy for individuals who have undergone gastric bypass surgery. Properly freezing and reheating meals ensures that gastric bypass patients have access to convenient, portion-controlled options that align with their post-surgery dietary guidelines. However, it's essential to follow safe handling practices to maintain food quality and prevent foodborne illness. This comprehensive guide will explore freezing and reheating guidelines specifically tailored for gastric bypass patients, including tips for safe storage, thawing, and reheating of frozen meals.

Freezing Guidelines:

Choose Suitable Containers: Use freezer-safe containers or bags designed for long-term storage to prevent freezer burn and maintain food quality.

Portion Control: Divide meals into individual or family-sized portions before freezing to facilitate portion control and prevent unnecessary waste.

Label and Date: Label each container with the name of the dish and the date it was prepared to track freshness and ensure timely consumption.

Cool Before Freezing: Allow cooked meals to cool completely before freezing to minimize condensation and prevent ice crystals from forming.

Freeze Quickly: Place cooked meals in the freezer promptly to freeze them as quickly as possible, reducing the risk of bacterial growth.

Avoid Overcrowding: Arrange frozen meals in the freezer in a single layer, leaving space between containers to allow for proper air circulation and faster freezing.

Use Proper Packaging: Wrap foods tightly in plastic wrap or aluminum foil before placing them in freezer-safe containers or bags to prevent freezer burn and maintain freshness.

Reheating Guidelines:

Thaw Safely: Thaw frozen meals in the refrigerator overnight or use the defrost setting on the microwave to thaw them safely. Steer clear of thawing at room temperature to stop the formation of microorganisms.

Microwave Reheating: Reheat individual portions of frozen meals in the microwave on high power until heated through, stirring halfway through cooking to ensure even heating.

Oven Reheating: For larger portions or meals with crispy textures, reheat in a preheated oven at a low temperature (around 300°F) until heated through, covering with foil to prevent drying out.

Stovetop Reheating: Reheat soups, stews, and sauces on the stovetop over medium heat, stirring frequently until heated through.

Check Temperature: Use a food thermometer to ensure that reheated meals reach a safe internal temperature of at least 165°F to kill any harmful bacteria.

Reheat Only Once: Avoid reheating meals multiple times to minimize the risk of bacterial contamination and maintain food quality.

Let Cool Before Consuming: Allow reheated meals to cool slightly before consuming to prevent burns and enjoy at a safe and comfortable temperature.

Considerations for Gastric Bypass Patients:

Portion Control: Use portioned containers to divide reheated meals into appropriate serving sizes, taking into account individual dietary needs and post-surgery restrictions.

Nutrient Retention: Option for gentle reheating methods such as microwave or stovetop to preserve the nutritional integrity of foods and prevent loss of essential nutrients.

Hydration: Drink water or other non-caloric beverages with meals to stay hydrated and support optimal digestion, especially when consuming reheated meals.

Listen to Your Body: Eat slowly to avoid pain or dumping syndrome, and pay attention to your body's signals of hunger and fullness. Even if there is food left on your plate, you should stop eating when you are full.

Portion Control Strategies

When it comes to eating a balanced diet and controlling weight, those who have had gastric bypass surgery must practice portion management. Patients undergoing gastric bypass surgery have a smaller stomach and a different digestive system, so it's important to watch portion sizes to avoid overindulging, pain, and problems.

Portion Control Strategies:

Use Portion-Controlled Containers:
Invest in portion-controlled containers or plates with designated compartments to visually guide

appropriate portion sizes for proteins,
carbohydrates, and vegetables.
Choose containers with clear markings or dividers
to help gauge portion sizes accurately and prevent
overfilling.

Measure Portions:
Use measuring cups, spoons, or a food scale to
measure ingredients and portion sizes when
preparing meals and snacks.
Familiarize yourself with recommended portion
sizes for different food groups, such as protein,
carbohydrates, fruits, and vegetables, to guide
portion control.

Follow the Plate Method:
Divide your plate into sections to ensure a balanced
meal that includes lean protein, non-starchy
vegetables, and a small portion of carbohydrates.

Fill half of your plate with vegetables, one-quarter with protein, and one-quarter with whole grains or starchy vegetables.

Visualize Serving Sizes:
When measurement equipment is not available, estimate proper portion sizes using visual clues. A portion of grains should be around the size of a tennis ball, a serving of vegetables should be about the size of your fist, and a serving of protein should be roughly the size of a deck of cards.

Practice Mindful Eating:
Pay attention to hunger and fullness cues, and eat slowly to allow time for your brain to register satiety signals.
Chew food thoroughly and savor each bite, focusing on the taste, texture, and aroma of the food to enhance satisfaction and prevent overeating.

Avoid Distractions:
Minimize distractions such as television, phones, or computers while eating to focus on your meal and prevent mindless eating.

Sit down at a table to eat meals rather than eating on the go or while multitasking to promote mindful eating and portion control.

Pre-Portion Snacks:
Divide snacks into individual portions in advance to prevent overindulging from large containers.
Choose nutrient-dense snacks such as raw vegetables with hummus, Greek yogurt with fruit, or a small handful of nuts to satisfy cravings without excess calories.

Be Mindful of Liquid Calories:
Limit consumption of high-calorie beverages such as sugary sodas, fruit juices, and alcoholic drinks, which can contribute to excess calorie intake and hinder weight management efforts.
Option for calorie-free beverages such as water, herbal tea, or sparkling water to stay hydrated without adding extra calories.

Considerations for Gastric Bypass Patients:

Protein Priority:

Prioritize consuming protein-rich foods to meet nutritional needs, support muscle maintenance, and promote satiety.
Ensure that each meal and snack includes a source of lean protein to support post-surgery recovery and weight management.

Hydration:
Between meals, keep hydrated and avoid dehydration, which can alter hunger signals and cause overeating. Instead, sip water or other non-caloric liquids.

Work with a Healthcare Professional:
Consult with a registered dietitian or healthcare provider to develop personalized portion control strategies tailored to your individual needs, preferences, and post-surgery dietary guidelines.

CHAPTER TEN

Managing Challenges and Plateaus

Gastric bypass surgery is a life-changing procedure that can lead to significant weight loss and improvements in overall health. However, like any weight loss journey, individuals may encounter challenges and plateaus along the way. Understanding how to manage these challenges

effectively is crucial for long-term success
post-surgery.

Common Challenges and Plateaus:

Stalled Weight Loss:
Plateaus in weight loss are common after gastric
bypass surgery, typically occurring around 6-12
months post-surgery.
Factors contributing to stalled weight loss may
include metabolic adaptations, changes in eating
habits, or decreased physical activity levels.

Nutritional Deficiencies:
Gastric bypass surgery can impact nutrient
absorption, leading to deficiencies in essential
vitamins and minerals such as vitamin B12, iron,
calcium, and vitamin D.
Inadequate nutrient intake can result from restrictive
dietary habits, poor supplement adherence, or
malabsorption issues.

Emotional Eating:
Gastric bypass patients may find it difficult to
control their emotional eating since they may use
food as a coping method for boredom, stress, or

worry. Emotional triggers can cause overindulgence in food or poor eating habits, which can impede the process of losing weight and exacerbate emotions of shame or guilt.

Body Image Concerns:
Significant weight loss following gastric bypass surgery may lead to changes in body image and self-esteem.
Patients may struggle with accepting their new body shape or experience body dysmorphia, which can impact mental well-being and overall quality of life.

Food Intolerances and Sensitivities:
Gastric bypass surgery can alter digestion and tolerance to certain foods, leading to intolerances or sensitivities.
Common triggers may include high-fat, high-sugar, or carbonated foods, which can cause gastrointestinal discomfort or dumping syndrome.

Strategies for Overcoming Challenges and Plateaus:

Seek Support:

Join a support group or seek guidance from a healthcare professional, registered dietitian, or therapist who specializes in bariatric surgery to address emotional, nutritional, and behavioral challenges.

Focus on Nutrient-Rich Foods:
Prioritize consuming nutrient-dense foods such as lean protein, fruits, vegetables, whole grains, and dairy products to meet nutritional needs and support overall health.

Monitor Portion Sizes:
Practice portion control strategies such as using smaller plates, measuring food portions, and following recommended serving sizes to prevent overeating and promote weight loss.

Develop Healthy Coping Mechanisms:

Find alternative coping mechanisms for managing stress or emotions, such as physical activity,

mindfulness meditation, journaling, or seeking
support from friends and family.

Stay Active:
Incorporate regular physical activity into your
routine, aiming for at least 150 minutes of
moderate-intensity exercise per week to support
weight loss, improve cardiovascular health, and
boost mood.

Adjust Eating Habits:
Focus on mindful eating, chewing food thoroughly,
eating slowly, and stopping when satisfied to
prevent overeating and promote better digestion.

Stay Consistent with Supplements:
Follow your healthcare provider's recommendations
for vitamin and mineral supplementation to prevent
deficiencies and support optimal health
post-surgery.

Address Body Image Concerns:
Seek support from mental health professionals or
support groups to address body image concerns,
develop self-compassion, and cultivate a positive
body image.

Maintaining Motivation and Momentum:

Set Realistic Goals:
Set achievable short-term and long-term goals for weight loss, health, and well-being to maintain motivation and track progress over time.

Celebrate Non-Scale Victories:
Acknowledge and celebrate non-scale victories such as improved energy levels, increased physical fitness, clothing size changes, or improvements in overall health markers.

Practice Self-Compassion:
Recognize that obstacles and disappointments are a normal part of the weight reduction process and treat yourself with kindness. Be kind to yourself and concentrate on making progress rather than perfection.

Stay Connected:

Stay connected with supportive friends, family members, or peers who understand your journey and can provide encouragement, accountability, and motivation when needed.

Dealing with Food Cravings

Food cravings can pose a challenge for individuals who have undergone gastric bypass surgery, as they may trigger overeating, unhealthy food choices, and feelings of guilt or frustration. Understanding how to manage food cravings effectively is crucial for maintaining weight loss, supporting nutritional goals, and promoting overall well-being post-surgery. In order to encourage long-term success, this thorough book will examine frequent causes for food cravings following gastric bypass surgery, hunger management techniques, and advice for creating a positive relationship with food.

Common Triggers for Food Cravings:

Emotional Triggers:
Stress, anxiety, boredom, sadness, or loneliness can trigger food cravings as individuals may seek comfort or distraction through eating.

Environmental Cues:
Exposure to food-related stimuli such as food advertisements, restaurant menus, or the sight and smell of food can trigger cravings, even in the absence of hunger.

Nutrient Deficiencies:
Following gastric bypass surgery, nutritional deficits may result in desires for particular foods that make up for the nutrients lost. For example,

low blood sugar levels may cause cravings for sweets, while electrolyte imbalances may cause cravings for salty foods.

Habitual Eating Patterns:
Established eating habits or routines, such as snacking while watching TV or indulging in dessert after dinner, can trigger cravings out of habit rather than true hunger.

Psychological Factors:
Memories, associations, or learned behaviors related to specific foods or eating occasions can trigger cravings, such as nostalgic childhood foods or favorite comfort foods.

Strategies for Managing Food Cravings:

Identify Triggers:
Recognize and identify the triggers for your food cravings, such as emotions, environmental cues, nutrient deficiencies, habits, or psychological factors.

Practice Mindfulness:

Increase awareness of your thoughts, feelings, and physical sensations surrounding food cravings through mindfulness practices such as deep breathing, meditation, or mindful eating.

Distract Yourself:
Redirect your attention away from food cravings by engaging in distracting activities such as going for a walk, practicing a hobby, listening to music, or calling a friend.

Address Underlying Emotions:
Explore the underlying emotions or stressors that may be driving your food cravings and develop alternative coping mechanisms for managing emotions, such as journaling, talking to a therapist, or practicing relaxation techniques.

Choose Nutrient-Dense Alternatives:
Option for nutrient-dense alternatives to satisfy cravings while supporting nutritional goals, such as choosing fruit for sweetness, nuts for crunchiness, or Greek yogurt for creaminess.

Practice Moderation:

Allow yourself to enjoy small portions of your favorite foods occasionally without guilt or restriction, practicing moderation and mindful eating to prevent overindulgence.

Plan Ahead:
Plan and prepare healthy meals and snacks in advance to prevent impulsive food choices and ensure that nutritious options are readily available when cravings strike.

Seek Support:
Reach out to a support group, therapist, or registered dietitian who specializes in bariatric surgery for guidance and support in managing food cravings and developing a healthy relationship with food.

Developing a Healthy Relationship with Food:

Focus on Nutritional Needs:
Prioritize consuming nutrient-dense foods that support your nutritional needs and promote overall health, emphasizing lean protein, fruits, vegetables, whole grains, and healthy fats.

Practice Intuitive Eating:
Tune into your body's hunger and fullness cues,
eating when hungry and stopping when satisfied,
rather than relying on external cues or emotional
triggers to dictate your eating patterns.

Cultivate Self-Compassion:
Be kind to yourself and practice self-compassion
when experiencing food cravings, recognizing that
cravings are a normal part of the human experience
and do not define your worth or success.

Experiment with Flavorful Options:
Explore new flavors, textures, and culinary
techniques to make nutritious foods more enjoyable
and satisfying, finding creative ways to incorporate
variety into your meals and snacks.

Overcoming Weight Loss Plateaus

Weight loss plateaus are common occurrences on
the journey after gastric bypass surgery. While
initially, significant weight loss is often observed,
progress may slow down or stall over time.
Understanding how to overcome these plateaus is
essential for continued success in achieving and

maintaining weight loss goals post-surgery. This guide will explore effective strategies for overcoming weight loss plateaus after gastric bypass surgery, including dietary adjustments, lifestyle modifications, and behavioral changes.

Reassess Your Diet:

Assess your eating patterns at the moment and decide where you can make changes. Make sure you are according to the post-operative dietary recommendations, which include getting enough protein, avoiding sweets and high-fat meals, and giving nutrient-dense foods priority.
Consider tracking your food intake using a food diary or mobile app to monitor portion sizes, calorie intake, and macronutrient distribution. This can help identify any hidden sources of calories or areas where adjustments may be needed.

Focus on Protein:

Prioritize protein-rich foods in your diet, as they are essential for maintaining muscle mass, supporting satiety, and promoting weight loss post-surgery. Incorporate lean sources of protein such as poultry, fish, tofu, eggs, and legumes into your meals and snacks. Aim to consume protein with each meal to support metabolic function and prevent muscle loss.

Increase Physical Activity:
Incorporate regular physical activity into your routine to enhance calorie expenditure and support weight loss efforts.
Try to get in at least 150 minutes a week of moderate-to-intense aerobic activity, such dancing, swimming, cycling, or brisk walking. Incorporate strength training activities as well to increase muscle mass and speed up metabolism.

Modify Meal Frequency and Timing:
Experiment with meal frequency and timing to optimize hunger control and calorie intake throughout the day.

Consider spreading out your meals and snacks evenly throughout the day to prevent excessive hunger and overeating. Some individuals may find success with intermittent fasting or time-restricted eating patterns, but consult with a healthcare professional before making significant changes to your eating schedule.

Stay Hydrated:
Drink plenty of water throughout the day to stay hydrated and support optimal metabolism and digestion.
Aim to drink at least 64 ounces of water daily, and prioritize water-rich foods such as fruits and vegetables to help meet your fluid needs.

Manage Stress:
Chronic stress can negatively impact weight loss efforts by increasing cortisol levels and promoting emotional eating.
Incorporate stress-reduction techniques such as mindfulness meditation, deep breathing exercises, yoga, or relaxation techniques into your daily routine to manage stress and promote overall well-being.

Get Adequate Sleep:
Prioritize getting sufficient sleep each night, as inadequate sleep can disrupt hormone levels, increase appetite, and sabotage weight loss efforts.

Aim for 7-9 hours of quality sleep per night and establish a regular sleep schedule to support optimal health and weight management.

Seek Support:
Reach out to your healthcare team, including your bariatric surgeon, dietitian, or support group, for guidance and support in overcoming weight loss plateaus.
Joining an online forum or bariatric support group might help you meet people who have gone through similar things and exchange tips for overcoming obstacles while trying to lose weight.

Seeking Support and Accountability

Seeking support and accountability is essential for individuals undergoing the transformative journey of gastric bypass surgery. Establishing a support system can provide encouragement, guidance, and accountability, helping individuals navigate challenges, celebrate successes, and stay motivated on their weight loss journey.

Importance of Seeking Support and Accountability:

Emotional Support:
The emotional journey of weight loss surgery can be challenging, with individuals experiencing a range of emotions, including excitement, anxiety, and uncertainty. Having a support system in place can provide emotional support, empathy, and understanding during difficult times.

Practical Guidance:
Support from healthcare professionals, such as bariatric surgeons, dietitians, and therapists, can provide practical guidance, education, and resources to help individuals navigate the post-surgery lifestyle changes effectively.

Motivation and Encouragement:
Encouragement and motivation from peers, family members, or support groups can inspire individuals to stay committed to their weight loss goals,

overcome obstacles, and celebrate achievements
along the way.

Accountability:

Accountability partners or groups can hold
individuals accountable for their actions, helping
them stay on track with dietary, exercise, and
lifestyle goals. Knowing that others are invested in
their success can increase motivation and adherence
to healthy behaviors.

Strategies for Building a Support Network:

Involve Family and Friends:

Share your weight loss journey with trusted family
members and friends, and enlist their support in
helping you achieve your goals. Communicate your
needs and boundaries, and ask for specific forms of
support, such as meal preparation, exercise buddies,
or emotional support.

Join a Support Group:

Seek out local or online support groups specifically
for individuals who have undergone gastric bypass
surgery. These groups provide a safe space to

connect with others who understand your experiences, share resources, and offer encouragement and advice.

Attend Follow-Up Appointments:
Stay engaged with your healthcare team by attending follow-up appointments with your bariatric surgeon, dietitian, and other specialists. These appointments provide opportunities to address concerns, track progress, and receive personalized guidance and support.

Connect with Peers:
Reach out to fellow gastric bypass patients who are at similar stages of their weight loss journey. Peer support can provide empathy, relatability, and practical tips for overcoming challenges and maintaining motivation.

Utilize Online Resources:
Explore online forums, social media groups, and websites dedicated to bariatric surgery and weight

loss. These platforms offer a wealth of information, community support, and success stories to inspire and motivate individuals on their journey.

Benefits of Accountability:

Increased Adherence:
Accountability fosters a sense of responsibility and commitment to following through with healthy behaviors, such as adhering to dietary guidelines, exercising regularly, and attending follow-up appointments.

Improved Consistency:
Knowing that others are monitoring your progress can increase consistency in adhering to healthy habits, even when motivation wanes or obstacles arise. Consistent effort over time leads to greater success in achieving weight loss goals.

Enhanced Motivation:
Accountability partners or groups provide encouragement, feedback, and reinforcement,

boosting motivation and confidence to overcome
challenges and persevere through setbacks.

Celebration of Achievements:
Accountability partners can celebrate successes and
milestones along the weight loss journey,
reinforcing positive behaviors and providing
encouragement to continue making progress.

Final Thoughts and Encouragement

Making the big choice to have gastric bypass
surgery calls for bravery, dedication, and fortitude.
Irrespective of whether you are contemplating

surgery, getting ready for the operation, or recovering from it, it is critical to embrace this life-changing experience with optimism and reasonable expectations. We provide some advice and motivation in this last section to help you on your journey to better health and wellbeing.

Embrace Your Strength:
Recognize the strength and courage it takes to pursue gastric bypass surgery as a tool for improving your health and quality of life. Your decision to prioritize your well-being is a powerful step towards a brighter and healthier future.

Stay Patient and Persistent:
Recognize that following gastric bypass surgery, the road to weight loss and recovery is not always straight-forward. Along the road, there could be achievements and failures, ups and downs. Remain patient with yourself and have faith in your capacity to persevere and conquer challenges.

Celebrate Small Victories
It's important to acknowledge and appreciate the minor successes and benchmarks you accomplish along the way, such as hitting a new weight reduction goal, adopting better eating habits, or

seeing enhancements in your general well-being and energy. Every stride you take ahead is evidence of your development and tenacity.

Practice Self-Compassion:
Throughout the process, treat yourself with kindness and care. Recognize that change takes time and that it's acceptable to have periods of uncertainty or hardship. Recognize that you are doing the best you can with the tools and help at your disposal, so be gentle and compassionate with yourself.

Cultivate a Supportive Network:
Assemble a network of friends, family, medical professionals, and other gastric bypass patients who are sympathetic to your situation and who will support you through any ups and downs. They can offer you advice, understanding, and encouragement.

Focus on Non-Scale Victories:
While weight loss is often a primary goal of gastric bypass surgery, remember that health and well-being encompass more than just a number on

the scale. Celebrate improvements in energy levels, mobility, self-confidence, and overall quality of life as equally valuable achievements on your journey.

Stay Committed to Self-Care:
Make self-nurturing and self-care routines a priority. These activities will nurture your body, mind, and soul. This might entail cultivating awareness, taking regular exercise, feeding your body wholesome meals, getting enough sleep, and asking for help when you need it.

Believe in Yourself:
Have faith in your ability to overcome challenges, adapt to change, and create the life you desire. Trust in your inner strength, resilience, and capacity for growth, knowing that you have the power to create positive change in your life.

CONCLUSION

The journey of gastric bypass surgery is a profound and transformative experience that encompasses physical, emotional, and psychological dimensions. Throughout this comprehensive guide, we have explored various aspects of gastric bypass surgery, including its benefits, dietary considerations, lifestyle changes, challenges, and strategies for success. From the initial decision to undergo surgery to the recovery process and long-term maintenance of health and well-being, each step of the journey is marked by courage, commitment, and resilience.

Gastric bypass surgery offers individuals struggling with obesity a powerful tool for achieving significant and sustainable weight loss, improving overall health, and enhancing quality of life. By reducing stomach capacity and altering the digestive process, gastric bypass surgery facilitates weight loss by limiting food intake, promoting satiety, and altering hormonal responses related to hunger and metabolism.

Additionally, the procedure can lead to improvements in obesity-related health conditions such as type 2 diabetes, hypertension, and sleep apnea, offering individuals a new lease on life and a renewed sense of vitality.

However, the journey of gastric bypass surgery is not without its challenges. From adjusting to dietary restrictions and lifestyle changes to navigating emotional and psychological hurdles, individuals may encounter obstacles along the way. These challenges may include adapting to new eating habits, managing food cravings, overcoming weight loss plateaus, and addressing body image concerns. Yet, with determination, perseverance, and support, individuals can overcome these challenges and emerge stronger, healthier, and more resilient than ever before.

Seeking support and accountability is essential for success on the journey of gastric bypass surgery. Whether it's leaning on family and friends for encouragement, connecting with fellow patients in support groups, or relying on healthcare

professionals for guidance and expertise, having a strong support network can make all the difference.

Additionally, cultivating self-compassion, celebrating victories, and staying committed to self-care are integral aspects of navigating the ups and downs of the weight loss journey with grace and resilience.

People undergoing gastric bypass surgery should keep in mind that the goal is to embrace a healthier, happier, and more rewarding life rather than merely reaching a specific weight on the scale. By using their inner strength, getting help, and remaining dedicated to their health and wellbeing, people may embrace the life-changing promise of gastric bypass surgery and reach their full potential. They get stronger and more capable of living life to the fullest with every step they take toward a better and healthier future.

We appreciate you looking over our cookbook about gastric bypass surgery! You're taking a revolutionary step towards becoming a better, happier version of yourself as you open these pages and go beyond simply accepting a cookbook. Your resolve to succeed is fueled by every meal, which not only nourishes your body but also your soul. We appreciate being on your journey to wellness because it motivates us to strive for personal improvement. Cheers to a tasty, rewarding future filled with food! Happy cooking!